Kyra's
Canine Conditioning

Peak Performance • Injury Prevention • Coordination • Flexibility • Rehabilitation

CANINE FITNESS EXPERT

NEW YORK TIMES BEST-SELLING AUTHOR

KYRA SUNDANCE

QUARRY

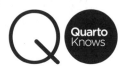

Inspiring | Educating | Creating | Entertaining

First Published in 2019 by Quarry Books, an imprint of The Quarto Group, 100 Cummings Center, Suite 265-D, Beverly, MA 01915, USA.
T (978) 282-9590 F (978) 283-2742 QuartoKnows.com

Quarry Books titles are also available at discount for retail, wholesale, promotional, and bulk purchase. For details, contact the Special Sales Manager by email at specialsales@quarto.com or by mail at The Quarto Group, Attn: Special Sales Manager, 100 Cummings Center, Suite 265-D, Beverly, MA 01915, USA.

10 9 8 7 6 5 4 3 2 1

ISBN: 978-1-63159-671-1

Digital edition published in 2019

Library of Congress Cataloging-in-Publication Data available

Design: Kyra Sundance
Expert Review: Cindy Otto DVM, Meghan Ramos VMD, Regina R. Allen DVM
Assistant Trainer: Rob Clark
Photography: Christian Arias, Shutterstock.com

Printed in China

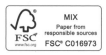

MIX
Paper from
responsible sources
FSC® C016973

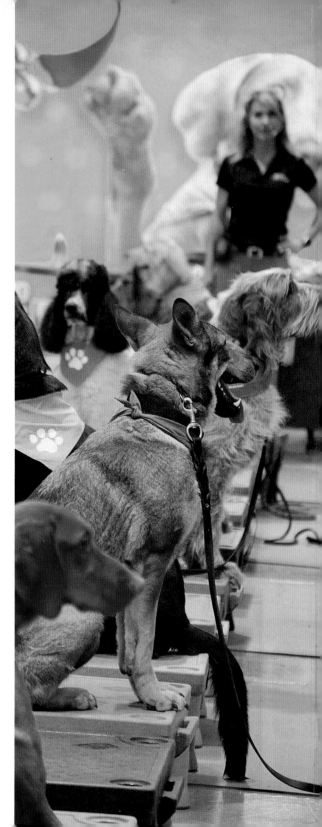

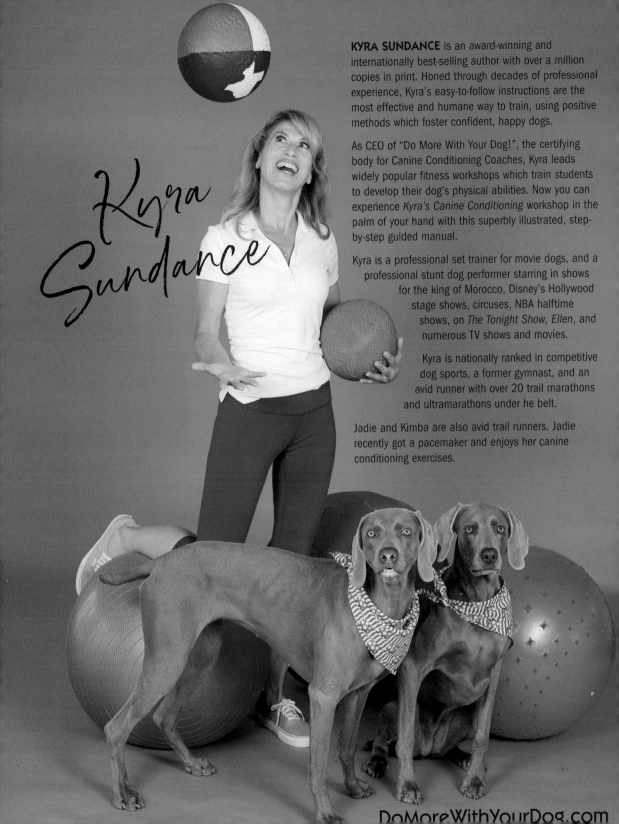

KYRA SUNDANCE is an award-winning and internationally best-selling author with over a million copies in print. Honed through decades of professional experience, Kyra's easy-to-follow instructions are the most effective and humane way to train, using positive methods which foster confident, happy dogs.

As CEO of "Do More With Your Dog!", the certifying body for Canine Conditioning Coaches, Kyra leads widely popular fitness workshops which train students to develop their dog's physical abilities. Now you can experience *Kyra's Canine Conditioning* workshop in the palm of your hand with this superbly illustrated, step-by-step guided manual.

Kyra is a professional set trainer for movie dogs, and a professional stunt dog performer starring in shows for the king of Morocco, Disney's Hollywood stage shows, circuses, NBA halftime shows, on *The Tonight Show*, *Ellen*, and numerous TV shows and movies.

Kyra is nationally ranked in competitive dog sports, a former gymnast, and an avid runner with over 20 trail marathons and ultramarathons under he belt.

Jadie and Kimba are also avid trail runners. Jadie recently got a pacemaker and enjoys her canine conditioning exercises.

Kyra Sundance

DoMoreWithYourDog.com

CONTENTS

LEVEL I

LEVEL II

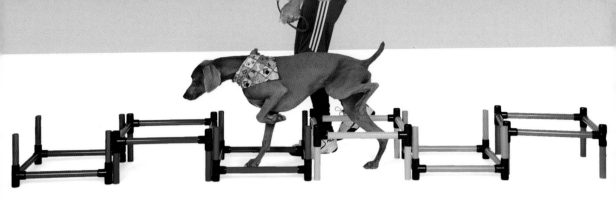

LEVEL III

LEVEL IV

Introduction

Physical fitness is just as important for dogs as it is for people. Improving a dog's fitness and health can increase their lifespan and limit vet visits as they get older. It reduces their risk of sports-related injury, joint problems, and arthritis. Dogs who are conditioned and healthy tend to live happier and more playful lives.

Exercise benefits a dog at every life stage. Puppies can improve their coordination, confidence, and mental focus while senior dogs can work on their strength and balance.

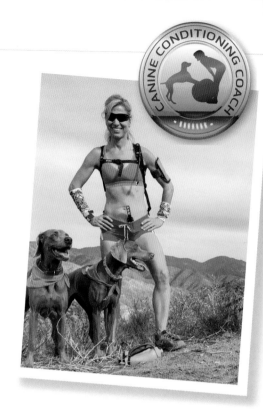

KYRA'S CANINE CONDITIONING WORKSHOPS

Kyra's world-renowned books and dog training programs have reached over a million people worldwide. An athlete herself, Kyra's passion for canine fitness led her to develop the widely popular Canine Conditioning Coach workshops which instruct dog owners on correct, safe, and enjoyable techniques for improving their dog's fitness.

Now, you can get this same knowledge in the palm of your hand, with this book.

A GUIDED STRATEGY OF CONDITIONING

This book is split into four levels of increasing difficulty. Each level builds upon previous skills with exercises that have been vetted to be effective and safe. Learn innovative ways to work with props such as hoops, balls, inflatables, and ladders as your dog improves in five components of fitness: flexibility, balance, stamina, coordination, and strength. Step-by-step instructions and photos are easy to follow and to execute.

Give your dog a new leash on life and turn the page to fitness!

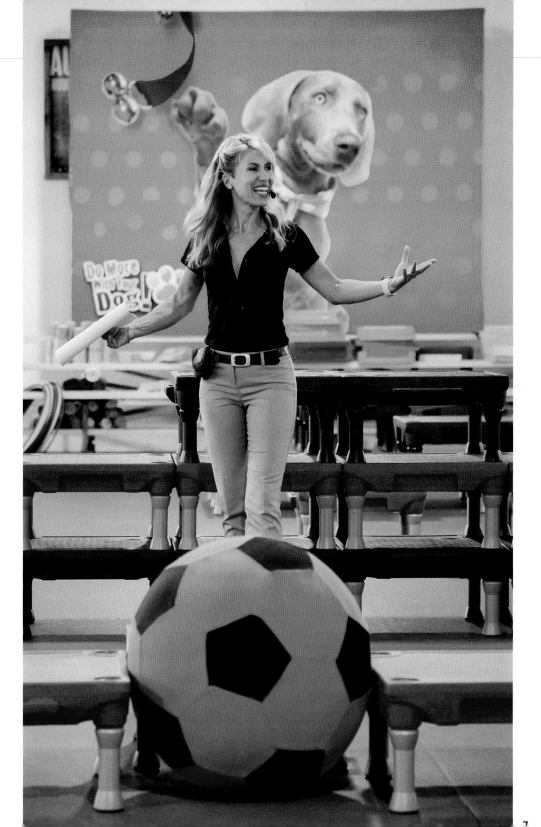

The 5 Fitness Components

A physically fit dog is conditioned in five areas. As canine conditioning coaches, we look at fitness as a whole, addressing each of the components with targeted exercises.

Many exercises demonstrated in this book will benefit more than one of the fitness components at the same time.

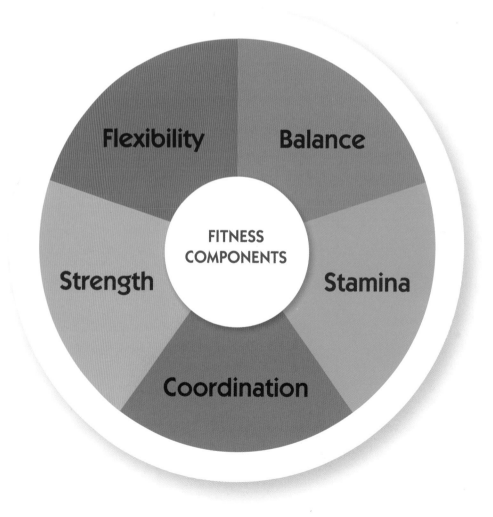

Flexibility

Balance

FITNESS COMPONENTS

Strength

Stamina

Coordination

FLEXIBILITY

Flexibility is the ability to move joints through a complete range of motion. We increase a dog's flexibility through stretching exercises that lengthen the muscles.

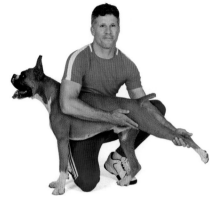

BALANCE

Balance is the dog's ability to evenly distribute his weight in order to remain upright and steady. It aids in injury prevention and is a strengthening technique in Instability Training.

STAMINA

Stamina (also called cardio) is a dog's ability to remain active for a long period of time, such as by jogging. Increasing endurance decreases anxiety and stress and reduces chronic diseases.

COORDINATION

Proprioception (also called coordination) is sometimes called our sixth sense. It is our ability to know where our body parts are, even in a dark room. Proprioception is a key component in fitness therapy. It allows our dog to learn new motor skills, and develop muscle memory. Training can vastly improve this sense.

STRENGTH

Strength is short-term explosive power, such as jumping over a high hurdle. Strength training protects bone health and muscle mass and is especially important for senior dogs to combat age-related muscle loss.

Assessing the Dog

An assessment of a dog's physiology is not necessarily a judgment on the perfection of the dog. Some breeds have long, thin limbs designed for speed, while others have wide shoulders designed for strength. We strive to design conditioning plans that strengthen weak areas and benefit each dog's unique physiology. Abnormalities should be evaluated by a veterinarian.

DOG SKELETAL STRUCTURE

The skeletal system is the dog's structural foundation. It consists of bones, cartilage, ligaments, and tendons. Long bones have growth plates that produce cartilage, which is converted to bone as the dog grows. At puberty, this bone growth slows, and the growth plates close when the dog reaches physical maturity, allowing no further growth. We want to avoid repetitive motion and high impact exercises before the dog's growth plates have closed.

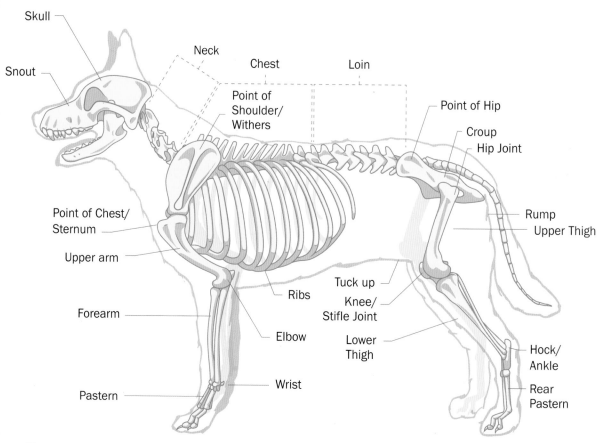

ANATOMIC STRUCTURE ZONES

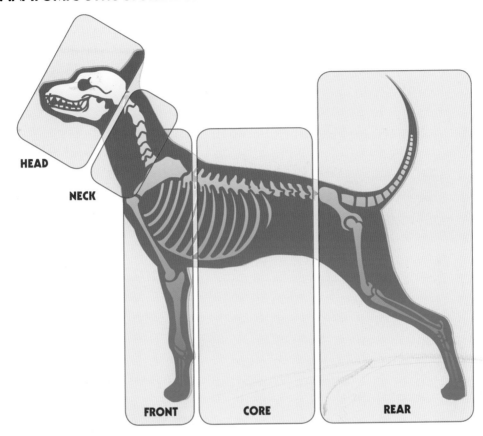

HEAD

NECK

FRONT **CORE** **REAR**

HEAD
There is a wide variety in head size and shape amongst different breeds.

NECK
The length of a dog's neck will affect his shoulders and spine.

FRONT
From the point of shoulder/withers down to the front paws, including the sternum.

CORE
Everything between the shoulder/ withers and the pelvis is known as a dog's core. A strong core supports the entire fitness of the dog.

REAR
The rear starts at the point of the hip and continues straight down and across to the rump of the dog.

Anatomy: Head

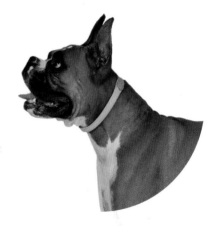

HEAD SIZE VS NECK SIZE

The head should be proportional to the neck. An oversized head can result in a dog with upper neck and back issues. These dogs can get exhausted faster.

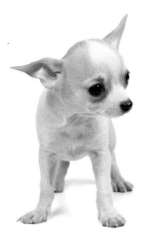

OVERSIZED HEAD
Common in teacup breeds such as large-headed Chihuahuas

NOSE

The nose provides ventilation to the dog. Dogs with flat noses (**brachycephalic** breeds) can have a hard time breathing and can overheat during exercise. Brachy dogs have an especially hard time running or going for long walks and have a tendency to overheat due to their snout shape. Swimming may be a good way for brachy breeds to get some cardio while staying cool.

FLAT NOSE/BRACHYCEPHALIC
Common in brachy dogs such as pugs, bulldogs, and boxers

Anatomy: Neck

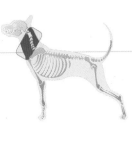

NECK LENGTH

The length of the dog's neck should be approximately the length of the dog's bottom jaw bone, but varies by breed and should be in proportion to the dog's body.

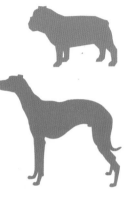

SHORT NECK / STIFF NECK

A short neck can lead to shoulder, back, and lower neck problems. A short neck is common in Labs, golden retrievers, spaniels, and bully breeds.

LONG NECK

A long neck, common in sighthounds, is vulnerable to being weak, resulting in neck and spine issues.

NECK ANGLE

The neck should be fairly straight and round slightly near the head. An excessively curved neck, where the whole neck rounds into the head, can result in a weak neck. A flat neck, or inverted rounding (like a swayback) neck can also result in a weak neck structure.

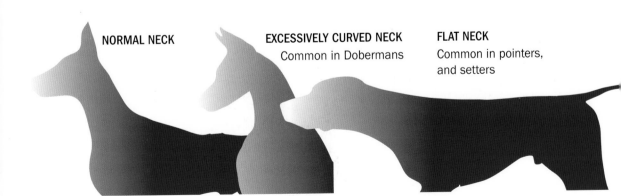

NORMAL NECK

EXCESSIVELY CURVED NECK
Common in Dobermans

FLAT NECK
Common in pointers, and setters

Anatomy: Front

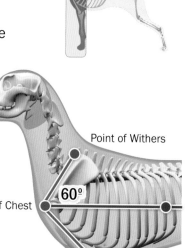

CHEST

There should be a 60-degree angle between the point of the withers to the point of the chest.

A **straight front** is characterized by the sternum tucked into the chest, and limits movement. When fronts are too straight it promotes arthritis in the shoulder, elbow, wrists, and feet (especially in an agility dog which lands repeatedly on a straight front).

Overangulation looks like a pointy chest. This condition is less common and creates an overall weak front.

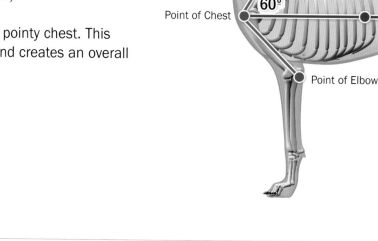

Point of Withers

Point of Chest

60º

Point of Elbow

FRONT ANGULATION

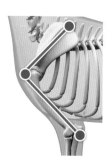

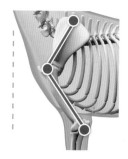

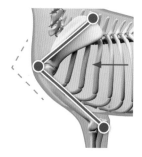

PERFECT

TOO STRAIGHT
Common in sighthounds and some terriers

TOO ANGULATED
Can appear in extra large breeds

SHOULDERS

Shoulders should be set around the first chest vertebrae. The highest point of the shoulder blade is called the **withers**. Shoulders set too far back, is a sign of **overangulation**. This is problematic with impact on movement. In a **stiff front** the shoulders are too far forward, looking like an overly straight, stiff front.

FRONT LEGS

A dog's front legs should sit at proper shoulder–chest angulation. When the front leg is bent up, the wrist should sit right in line with the chest point. If not, it indicates that either the upper arm or the forearm are too long.

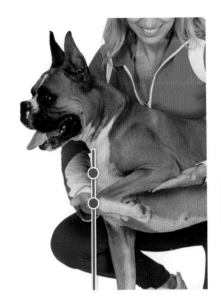

FEET

Trimming a dog's nails is important for his stance, and allows him to stand with correct posture. Notice how nice and arched the toes are on the foot with the freshly cut nails. Then look at the other foot. The toes are leaning forward because of the grossly long nails.

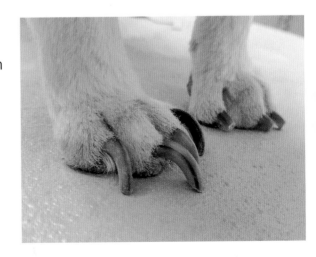

Anatomy: Core

TOPLINE

A dog's **topline** should be straight and parallel to the ground
or taper off slightly toward the rear. This can vary by breed.
A **roached** back is raised in the middle, and seen in German shepherds and
whippets. Roached backs can lead to an increase in injury, especially for active dogs.
A **swayback**, or high rear, is a back that is lower in the middle than in the rear. This
condition is sometimes seen in bully breeds and can result in back problems.

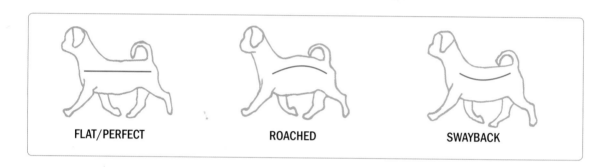

| FLAT/PERFECT | ROACHED | SWAYBACK |

LOIN

The loin is the distance between that last rib and the pelvis. A **long loin**, common in
dachshunds, corgis, and Bassett hounds, can result in a weak structure and back
problems especially for dogs that do repetitive jumping and landing. A **short loin**,
common in pomeranians and herding breeds, can result in limited flexibility.

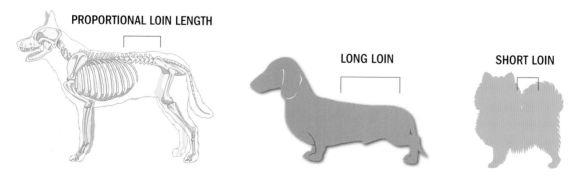

PROPORTIONAL LOIN LENGTH

LONG LOIN

SHORT LOIN

WEIGHT

Evaluate a dog's weight and shape as part of the overall assessment of their body condition. Overweight dogs will experience strain in all areas of their structure.

With an ideal weight, the dog's ribs will be easily palpable, with minimal fat covering. Their waist is apparent when viewed from above. Their abdominal tuck is evident when viewed from the side. The dog should have a slight **tuck up** after the end of the ribcage under the loin.

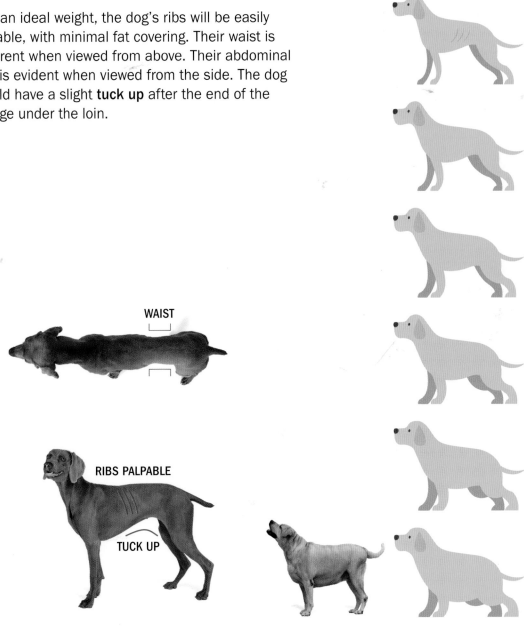

WAIST

RIBS PALPABLE

TUCK UP

Anatomy: Rear

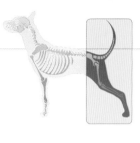

REAR LEGS

When the dog's hock is perpendicular to the ground, there should be approximately 90-degree angles between the highest hip point (iliac crest), the point of the rump (body ischium), and the knee (bony patella). Ideally, the toes should be behind the rear (can vary by breed).

When the hock is at a 90-degree angle, the toes are under dog. If any angle is greater than 100 degrees, the angulation is **too straight**. This condition will keep a dog from being able to leap effectively and is also associated with crucial rupture.

An **overangulated**, or weak rear, is when any angle is less than approximately 80 degrees. This condition puts strain on knees and hips and can lead to knee arthritis or recurring rear leg muscle strain.

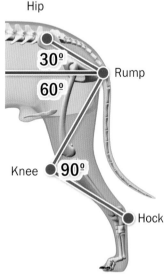

Hip

30º

Rump

60º

Knee 90º

Hock

REAR LEG ANGULATION

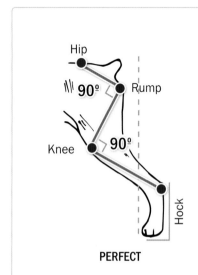

Hip

90º

Rump

Knee

90º

Hock

PERFECT

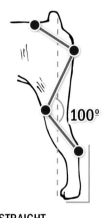

100º

TOO STRAIGHT

Common in bully breeds

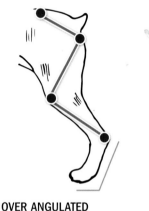

OVER ANGULATED

Common in poodles, northern breeds, and German shepherds.

HIPS

The hips should be able to stretch and move easily. You should be able to easily lift the dog's rear legs as indicated in the stretches on page 26. If the dog cannot complete stretches easily, this may indicate **stiffness**, limited flexibility, or hip dysplasia. This problem is common in older dogs and should be evaluated by a veterinarian.

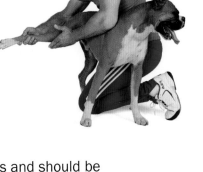

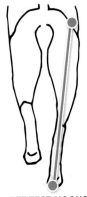

PERFECT HOCKS

HOCKS

When viewed from behind, hocks are even and straight in line with the rump and feet and converge toward the midline when trotting.

Cow hocked, common in bully breeds and some herding breeds, are when hocks are pointed inward. This condition can result in weaker hind legs, ineffective running, and difficulty jumping, which can lead to hip, rear leg, and back injury.

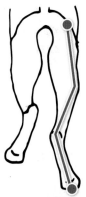

COW HOCKED

A **bow-legged** dog has hocks pointed outward. Bowed legs are common in bulldogs, Labs, and cattle dogs. This condition results in more hock and knee injuries during running and jumping, especially during jump take off.

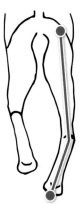

BOW LEGGED

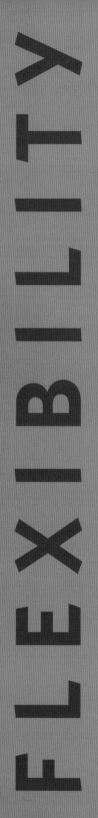

FLEXIBILITY

Flexibility exercises can improve your dog's posture, prevent muscular imbalances leading to injuries, and reduce soreness after a workout.

Stretching should be done on **warm muscles** not cold, stiff muscles. Warm up with a few minutes of jogging or moving before stretching. Stretching can also be done at the end of an exercise session, to loosen muscles and avoid cramping.

Stretching should feel mild and relaxing and not uncomfortable or painful. Signs your dog is feeling pain include

- Whining
- Whipping head back toward your arm, as if to bite
- Pulling back corners of lips; smiling
- Panting
- Licking lips
- Pulling leg away from you
- Whale eyes
- Pupils dilating

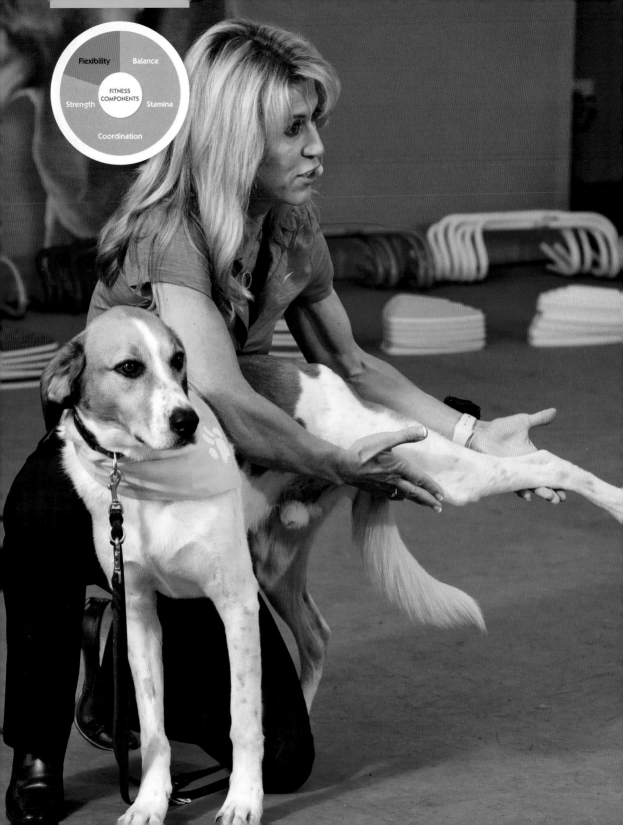

Flexibility Balance
FITNESS
COMPONENTS
Strength Stamina
Coordination

Passive Range of Motion

TECHNIQUE: PASSIVE RANGE OF MOTION (PROM)

BENEFIT: EXPANDS RANGE OF MOTION IN LIMBS

As dogs age, or when they are recovering from an injury, they may have reduced range of motion in their joints. This reduced mobility causes decreased blood flow and flexibility of the joints, which could become stiff and locked.

We use **Passive Range of Motion (PROM)** exercises on the dog to help keep joint areas flexible.

TARGET: Hind limbs, fore limbs, back, hips

REPEAT: 2–3 times per day

TIME: 1–2 minutes for each exercise

PROM exercises require no effort from the dog as you manually move their joints through their full range of motion. This will warm the joint fluid and improve blood flow to help joints and muscles feel more comfortable.

Perform these exercises at a time when your dog is relaxed and quiet. Start conservatively and slowly increase the range of motion.

PASSIVE RANGE OF MOTION EXERCISES

- Keep joint areas flexible
- Increase blood flow
- Warm joint fluid
- Alleviate stiffness

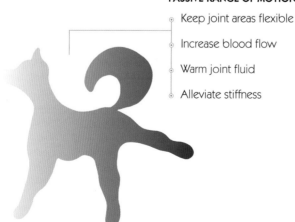

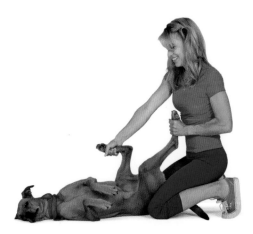

1. Move the knee and ankle joints through their range of motion by gently bicycling the legs.

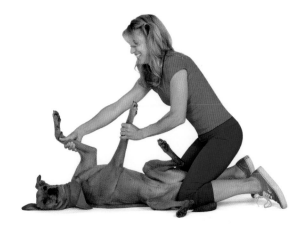

2. Bicycle the front limbs while avoiding putting significant tension on the muscles.

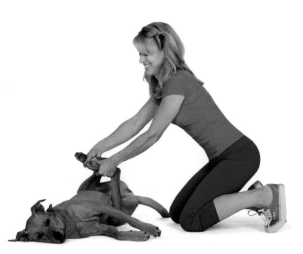

3. Twist the spine. Instead of holding the position, constantly move the hind legs so the spine twists and straightens again.

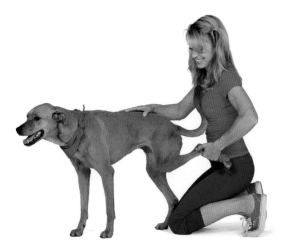

4. Lift the hind leg up to expand the hip, and back down again.

Static Stretch: Front Limbs

TECHNIQUE: STATIC STRETCHING, EXTENSION, FLEXION

BENEFIT: EXPANDS FRONT LEG RANGE OF MOTION

Stretching promotes increased range of motion, circulation, and increased oxygen to the dog's muscles.

Static stretching is a type of stretch whereby you stretch the muscle until a gentle tension is felt, and then hold the stretch. In static stretch, there is no movement or bouncing.

Don't rush the stretching. Watch your dog's reaction to your manipulation in order to gauge when he starts to feel discomfort (see page 20). If your dog pulls away, the stretch may be too aggressive, or the area may be sore. Never force a joint or muscle. Stop the stretch when you start to feel slight resistance, and hold the stretch there for 5–30 seconds.

Always hold the limb you are stretching with both hands. Open palms and gently cup the limb to avoid squeezing or stressing the joint.

Static stretching should be done after exercise, on warm muscles.

TARGET: Shoulder flexors and extensors, chest, biceps, triceps.

REPEAT: 2–3 times on each side

TIME: 5–30 seconds each repetition

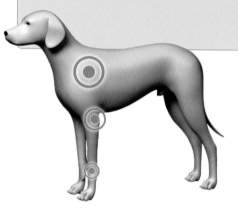

EXTENSION

Straightening the joint

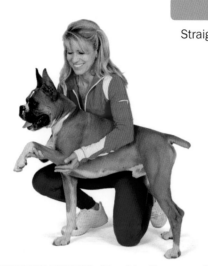

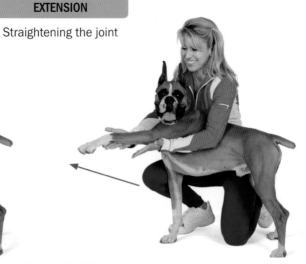

1. **SUPERMAN STRETCH:** Shoulder flexors and extensors enable smooth movement and proper use of your dog's front legs. Support the dog's wrist with one hand and the dog's elbow with the other.

2. With an open palm, gently press up on the elbow until you feel slight resistance. Hold for 5 to 30 seconds.

FLEXION

Bending the joint

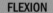

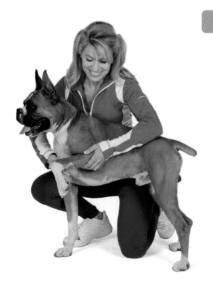

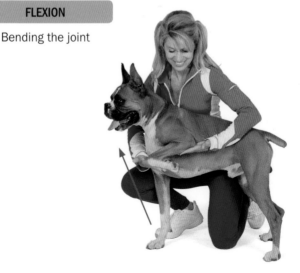

1. **SCRUNCH-UP STRETCH:** Support the dog's wrist and elbow.

2. With an open palm, gently press the dog's elbow up into his chest. Fold his wrist until you feel slight resistance. Hold for 5 to 30 seconds.

Static Stretch: Hind Limbs

TECHNIQUE: STATIC STRETCHING, EXTENSION, FLEXION, ABDUCTION

BENEFIT: EXPANDS HIND LIMB RANGE OF MOTION

Stretching is when a specific muscle or tendon (or muscle group) is deliberately flexed or stretched. Routine stretching increases muscle elasticity and control, flexibility, and range of motion. Stretching is also used to alleviate cramps.

As you stretch your dog, notice differences between his left and right limbs. A difference may indicate a problem with the limb you are currently manipulating, or it may indicate a problem standing on or balancing on the opposite limb. Imbalances should be evaluated by a veterinarian.

Hip flexors (iliopsoas) is a common injury in dogs who train in the sport of agility.

TARGET: Quads, hip flexors (iliopsoas), hamstrings, glutes, lower back muscles, gastrocnemius, and Achilles tendon.

REPEAT: 2–3 times on each side

TIME: 5–30 seconds each repetition

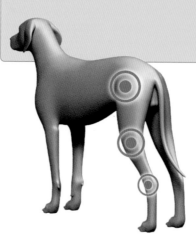

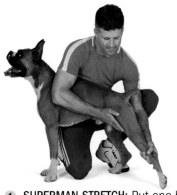

EXTENSION

Straightening the joint

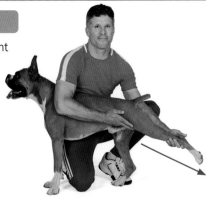

1 **SUPERMAN STRETCH:** Put one hand under the knee and the other on the hock. Do not grab or pull.

2 Support the hock, and press up on the knee until the dog's hock is just below his back.

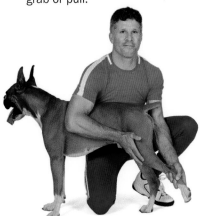

FLEXION

Bending the joint

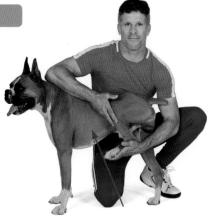

1 **SCRUNCH-UP STRETCH:** Put one hand under the knee and the other on the hock.

2 Scrunch the leg up into the dog's belly. Press on the knee and also on the hock.

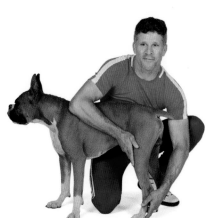

ABDUCTION

Moving a limb away from the center line of the body

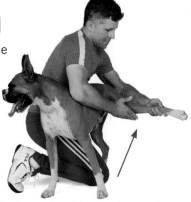

1 **LEG HIKE STRETCH :** Put one hand under the knee, and the other on the hock.

2 Lift the leg to the side, gently pressing upward on both the knee and the hock.

BALANCE

Balance is a complex system that requires mental and physical fitness. A dog depends on several body systems to keep upright. The inner ear, which senses head motions, plays an important role as does the proprioception system, which relays the feeling of the ground beneath his feet. And, of course, vision informs him of obstacles.

Tai chi, a form of human exercise that involves moving gently through a series of poses, improves our balance because it works with both the mind and body. In this chapter, we will be doing something similar to tai chi with our dog.

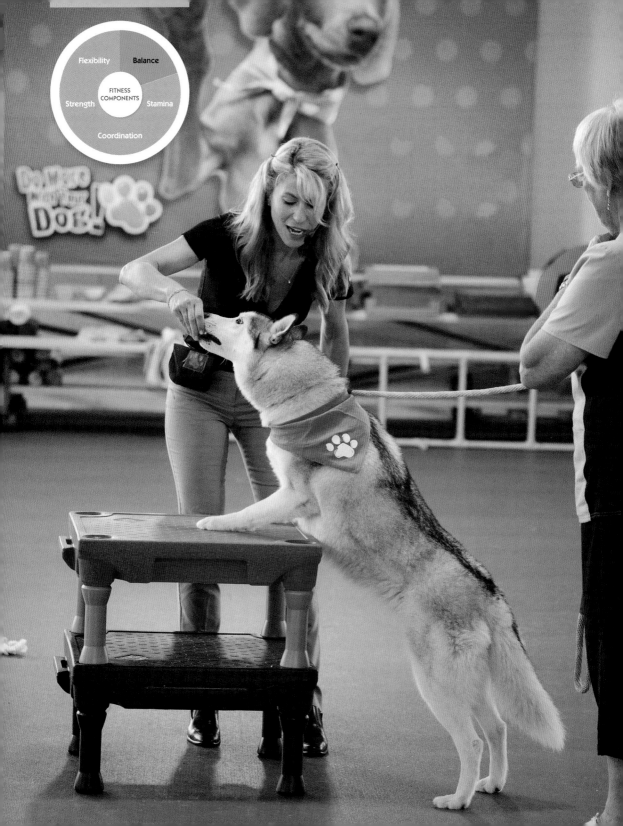

FITNESS COMPONENTS

Flexibility

Balance

Strength

Stamina

Coordination

Paws up on a Pedestal

TECHNIQUE:	STATIC BALANCE
BENEFIT:	STRENGTHENS CORE AND FOREARM MUSCLES

There are two types of balance: static and dynamic. **Static balance** is the ability of the dog to maintain his body in a fixed posture.

Your dog is used to maintaining his balance while standing on the floor, but in this exercise, he is challenged to maintain that balance with his front feet raised.

This exercise is about maintaining proper posture. Raise the height of the platform only when your dog is able to perform this exercise stably, and with proper form.

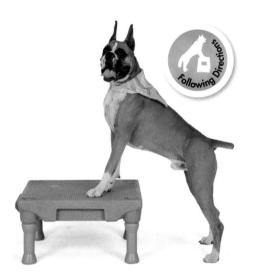

STATIC BALANCE REQUIRES

- Enough muscle in the lower limbs and trunk to maintain the body erect
- Postural sensibility to convey information concerning position
- Impulses from the vestibular labyrinth (inner ear) concerning position

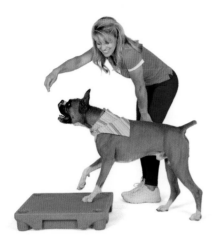

1. Set a low, sturdy platform. Use a treat to lure your dog to put his front feet on it.

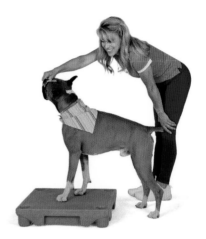

2. Give the dog the treat while he is still in the correct position (with front feet on the platform).

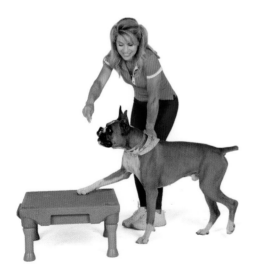

3. Raise the platform. Again, slowly move the treat from your dog's nose to over the center of the platform.

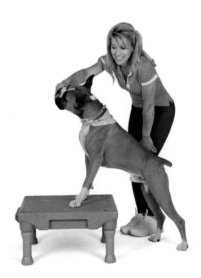

4. Allow your dog to nibble or lick a treat to keep him there. Shift the treat a little to cause your dog to readjust his balance.

Paws up on Balance Disc

TECHNIQUE:	DYNAMIC BALANCE/INSTABILITY TRAINING
BENEFIT:	IMPROVES BALANCE, STRENGTHENS CORE AND FOREARM MUSCLES

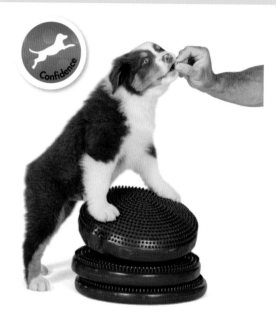

In the previous exercise, your dog used static balance. In this exercise, he will use **dynamic balance**, which is maintaining equilibrium while in motion or switching between positions.

Your dog uses his eyes, ears, and proprioception, or muscle sense, to help retain balance. Your dog will learn to use his proprioception and mind to quickly compensate for shifts in the object beneath his feet.

Have you ever stood on something that moved and made you slip, and caused you to feel a moment of panic? We want to avoid that situation with our dogs. Flat balance discs are fairly stable and will allow your dog to develop his confidence as well as muscle strength and balance.

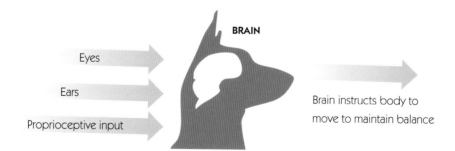

BRAIN

Eyes

Ears

Proprioceptive input

Brain instructs body to move to maintain balance

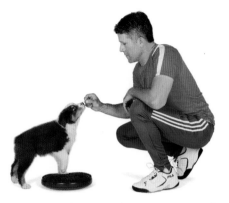

1 Use a treat to lure your dog to step on and off the balance disc.

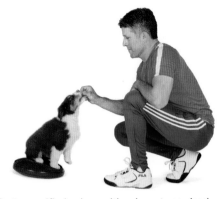

2 A specific body position is not required. Ask your dog for a "sit" on top of the disc.

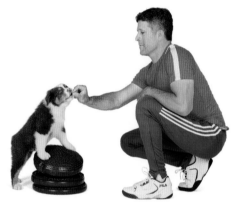

3 Make it more challenging by adding several balance discs. Progress only when your dog is able to maintain good posture.

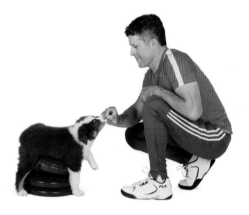

4 Your dog will gain confidence as he maneuvers this new game.

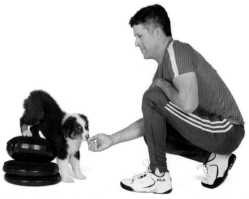

5 Keep luring the dog over the disc until his back feet are on it.

Fit Bones

TECHNIQUE: INSTABILITY TRAINING

BENEFIT: IMPROVES BALANCE, STRENGTHENS WHOLE BODY

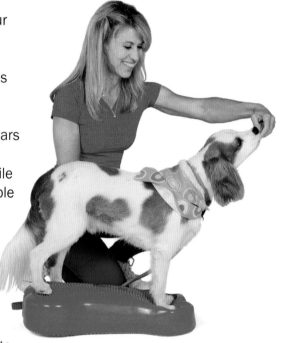

Training on unstable surfaces increases your dog's muscle activation, improves proprioception and balance, and improves neuromuscular control, all of which improves his functional performance.

A very popular mode of training in recent years has been the use of instability devices and exercises to train the core musculature. While struggling to maintain balance on an unstable object, the dog tightens his body.

Instability training requires high-intensity concentration from your dog, and this residual benefit will improve his mind and focus.

In this exercise, your dog will be introduced to instability training by learning to mount and dismount an inflatable fit bone, and to manage his balance while standing on the bone.

FULL BODY CONDITIONING

- Core and limb strength
- Coordination
- Joint health
- Mental focus
- Senior strengthening
- Puppy confidence
- Low-impact therapy

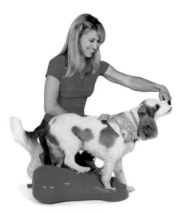

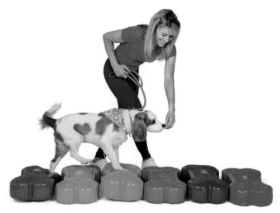

1 Use a treat to lure your dog to step on the squishy object.

2 Engage all four limbs by arranging a pathway of multiple fit bones. Hold the treat at nose height to keep his neck and back in line.

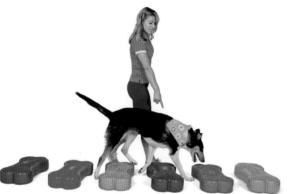

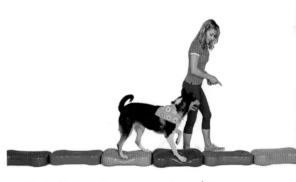

1 Adding spaces between bones will require your dog to constantly evaluate steady versus unstable foot placements.

2 A skinny rail arrangement requires lateral balance adjustments and shoulder activation.

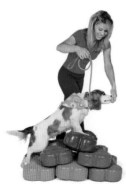

1 Three to five minutes of instability training will give your dog a surprisingly strenuous workout.

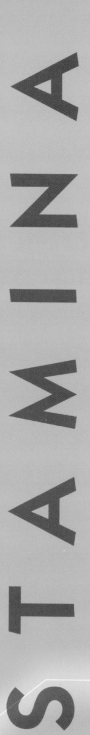

STAMINA

Aerobic exercise strengthens your dog's respiratory muscles (lungs) and heart. This will reduce blood pressure and increase red blood cells, facilitating transport of oxygen and resulting in athletic efficiency.

Endurance exercise also reduces anxiety and increases cognitive capacity.

Warm up Before each stamina workout session, warm up for 5 to 10 minutes to gradually rev up your dog's cardiovascular system and increase blood flow to his muscles. Try a low-intensity version of your planned activity.

Conditioning At your dog's pace, work up to 20 minutes of cardio to increase your dog's heart rate, depth of breathing, and muscle endurance.

Cool down After each session, cool down for 5 to 10 minutes by slowing down to a walk. This allows your dog's heart rate and muscles to return to normal.

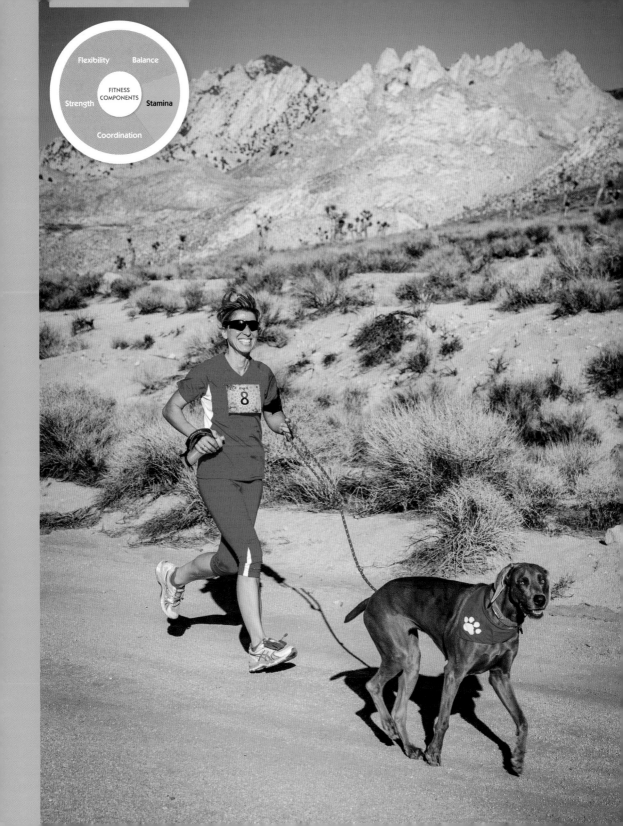

FITNESS COMPONENTS

Flexibility   Balance

Strength   Stamina

Coordination

Treadmill

TECHNIQUE:	RHYTHMIC MOVEMENT TRAINING
BENEFIT:	CARDIOVASCULAR STAMINA

In addition to evaluating our dog's physical structure while standing still, we want to also evaluate her structure in movement. A dog treadmill allows you to watch and evaluate your dog's gait and check for abnormalities.

Rhythmic Movement Training (RMT) is a system of gentle, rhythmic movements. RMT is used with children to improve attention, impulse control, brain connectivity, as well as physical strength and stamina.

Long-term endurance training leads to decreased heart rate, increased stroke volume of the heart, increased blood flow to muscles, and increased muscle tone. One of the best endurance training exercises you can provide for your dog is the extended trot gait on a treadmill. This weight-bearing exercise works both sides of the body evenly. Use a treadmill with a belt length of at least one and a half times the length of the dog. Work your way up to having your dog gait with a low to medium intensity for 20 minutes.

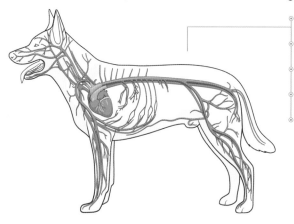

5 BENEFITS OF ENDURANCE ACTIVITY

⊙ Improves the aerobic capacity of muscles

⊙ Aids in weight loss

⊙ Improves sleep quality

⊙ Prevents age-related decline in brain function

⊙ Maintains good postural stabilization

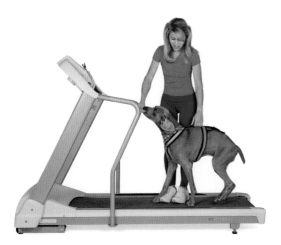

1 Introduce the treadmill to your dog when it is turned off. Stand on it yourself, and encourage her to explore it.

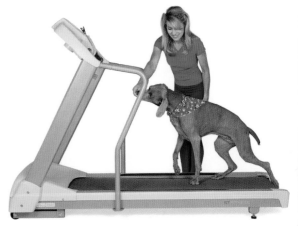

2 Set the treadmill to its slowest setting. Use a treat to lure your dog on from the rear.

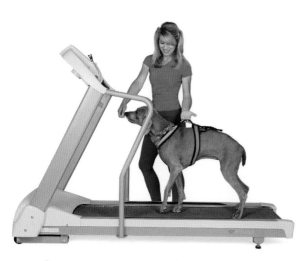

3 A harness will be helpful to keep your dog steady and not making sudden leaps off of the treadmill. Keep a light hand on the harness, but do not tether the dog to the treadmill.

COORDINATION

Motor coordination is the combination of body movements that result in intended actions. Often, several body parts or limbs are required to move in a way that is synchronized, well timed, smooth, and efficient.

Coordination is a complex skill that requires not only good balance but also strength and agility. It involves the integration of **proprioceptive** information (knowing where our body is in space) with brain signals telling our body where to move next.

Good coordination is important for excelling at most dog sports, especially ones that require quick changes in speed and direction. It can make your dog a better athlete, and less prone towards falling and injury.

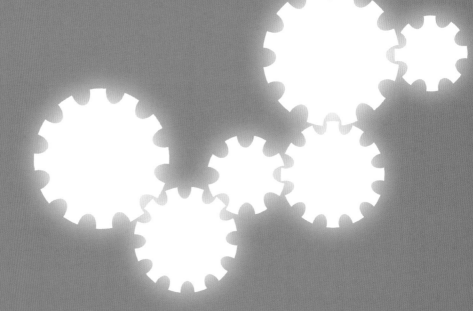

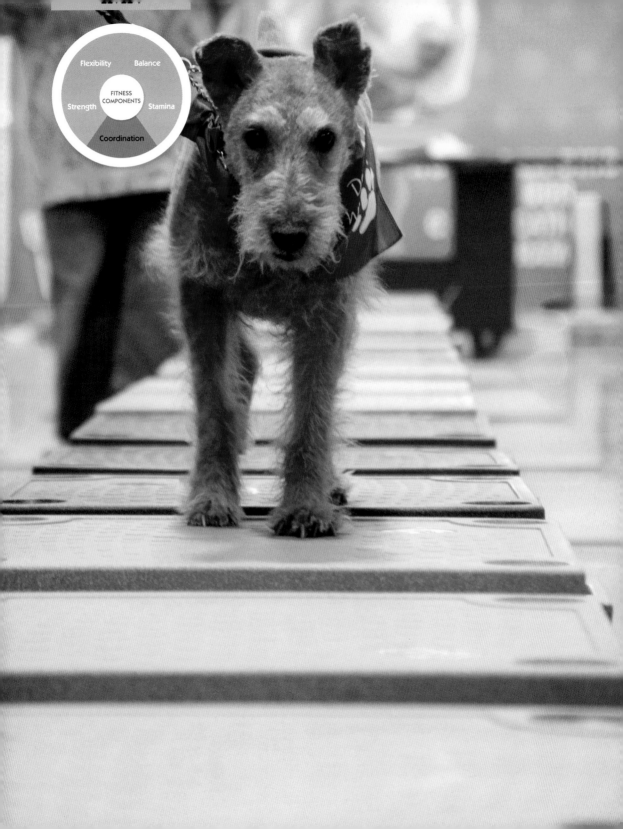

FITNESS COMPONENTS

Flexibility Balance
Strength Stamina
Coordination

Scattered Sticks

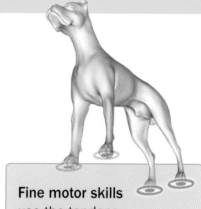

TECHNIQUE: AGILITY

BENEFIT: IMPROVE PROPRIOCEPTION/HIND-END AWARENESS

It is commonly joked that "dogs don't know they have back feet," as they seem to move along with their front feet, while their back feet just follow behind. Knowing how to specifically place those back feet is a skill that can be easily improved, and a skill that will help prevent injury (think of a search-and-rescue dog navigating over rubble or an agility athlete running the dog walk). This skill of knowing where your body parts are in space is called **proprioception**.

In this exercise, your dog will build his proprioception by walking through a yard of scattered poles. He will need to think about where he places each foot.

Fine motor skills use the tendons, ligaments, and small muscles of the dog's toes, ankles, and wrists.

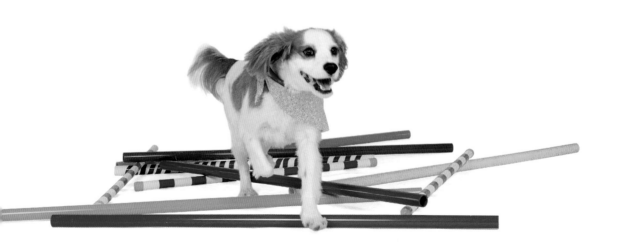

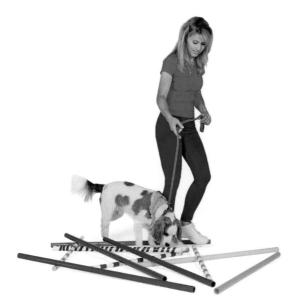

1 Scatter several poles (or other objects) on the ground. Use a leash to slowly walk your dog through them.

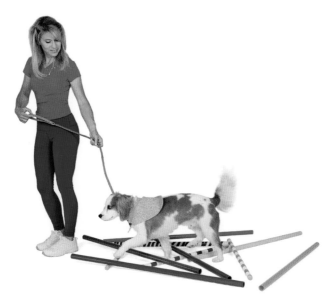

2 The first few times your dog walks through the poles, he may stumble with his back feet, but by the fifth time you should see him deliberately thinking about the placement of his back feet.

Walk Line of Platforms

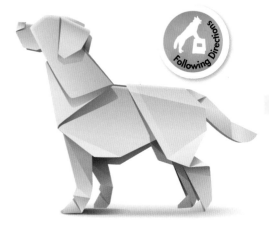

TECHNIQUE:	CONTINUOUS MOTOR SKILLS
BENEFIT:	GROSS MOTOR SKILLS

After your dog has had experience with floor-level exercises (previous page), we can work an elevated exercise. Exercises utilizing your dog's **gross motor skills** require coordinated movement of large muscle groups such as walking and running.

Walking and running exercises require coordination, but do not have a defined start and finish. These exercises are a type of **continuous motor skills**.

In this exercise, your dog will walk a line platforms. Challenge him further by staggering, rotating, and randomizing the platforms.

GROSS MOTOR-SKILL EXERCISES IMPROVE

- Core and limb strength
- Postural control
- Sensory processing
- Body awareness
- Balance
- Coordination
- Motor (muscle) planning

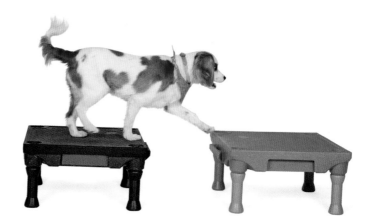

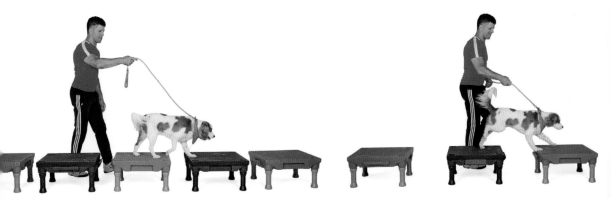

1. Construct a line of platforms for your dog to walk across. It is best to not use a treat lure in this exercise, as your dog will need to watch his feet. You may wish to leave a treat at the end of the line or simply hand him a treat at the end.

2. Gradually increase the space between platforms. Vary the space between each, to cause your dog to continually reassess his movements.

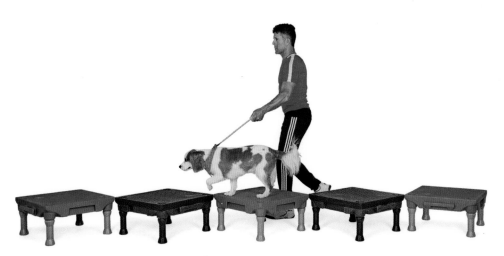

3. Set the platforms on angle or pull some out to the side. Allow your dog to go at his own pace.

Targeting: Nose Touch Your Hand

TECHNIQUE:	TARGETING
BENEFIT:	NOSE-EYE COORDINATION/DISCRETE MOTOR SKILLS

In this exercise, you dog will learn to nose-touch your open palm. This **targeting** skill will be used to move your dog into various body positions.

Nose-eye coordination skills require the ability of the dog to coordinate visual information and then navigate his nose to a specific spot. In humans, this would be called hand-eye coordination, which is used in tasks such as catching a ball, sewing, or using a computer mouse.

Discrete motor skills are skills that have an observable start and finish. So, for example, nose-touching your hand is a discrete movement. The dog aims, touches your hand, and it's done!

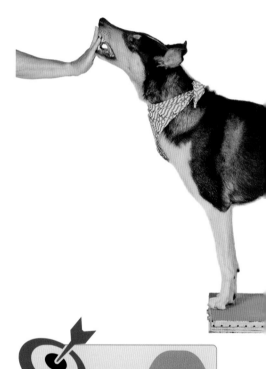

Targeting is a foundation skill of canine conditioning. It is used to draw the dog into a position or onto a piece of equipment. A dog can learn to touch a target with his nose, or with his front foot, rear foot, hip, or other body part.

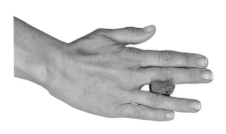

1 Hold a treat between your fingers.

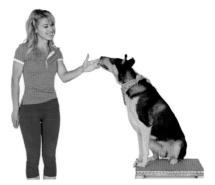

2 Hold you palm to your dog and say "touch!" Don't push your hand toward him, but make him come to you. Let him take the treat.

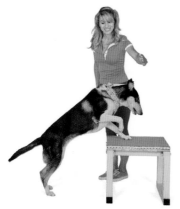

3 Once your dog understands your "touch" cue, use your hand as a target to get him to jump onto a pedestal.

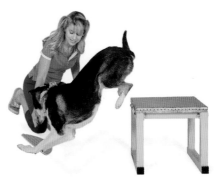

4 Hold your palm at the ground and use it as a target to get your dog to jump off the pedestal.

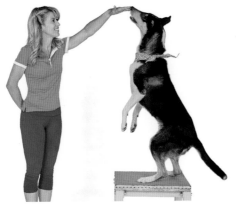

5 Have your dog target your hand up high for a core strength exercise.

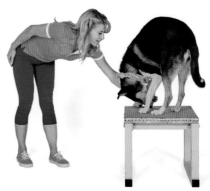

6 Place your target hand between his front paws for a neck/spine stretch.

Rainbow Ladder

TECHNIQUE:	RHYTHMIC MOVEMENT TRAINING
BENEFIT:	IMPROVE PROPRIOCEPTION/HIND-END AWARENESS

In the **scattered sticks** exercise (page 42), we made the dog think about where he is placing his back feet. In this exercise, we will build on that coordination skill by challenging him to rhythmically trot over ladder rungs.

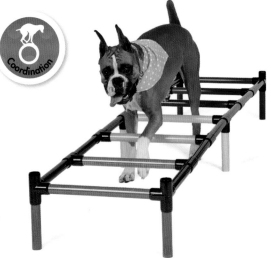

Ladder work is a foundation tool in dog sports, and in canine conditioning and rehabilitation.

The rainbow ladder exercise is designed to increase your dog's proprioception, coordination, and focus, and can be used in a variety of exercises.

MORE WAYS TO USE THE RAINBOW LADDER:

- Cavalettis (walk through it low)
- Stride regulators (trot through it high)
- Elevation change (ladder at an angle)
- Step backward through it
- Front feet only (dog walks to the side)
- Back feet only

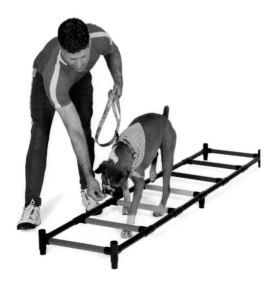

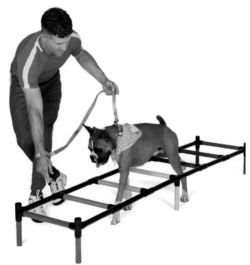

1. Start with a low ladder. Walk your dog slowly through it, on leash. If you need to use a treat, hold the treat low, near the rungs, so that your dog can see both the treat and the ladder.

2. Raise the ladder. Use your pointed finger, held low, to focus your dog forward.

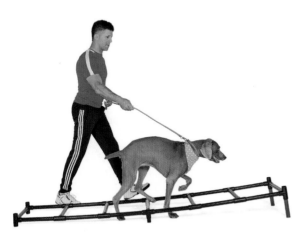

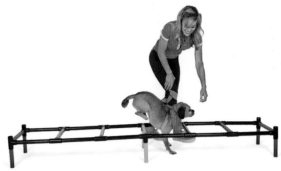

3. Try an angled ladder that starts low and increases in height.

4. Dogs will use different cadences. Some may bunny hop through the rungs.

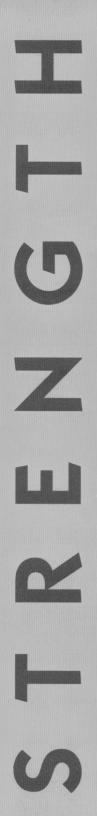

STRENGTH

Having good balance can prevent a dog from falling. But if the dog *does* lose balance, recovering requires muscle power.

Power is the ability to exert force quickly— such as to push off when jumping a bar jump. Rapid, forceful exercises like hopping and side stepping help to build power and agility.

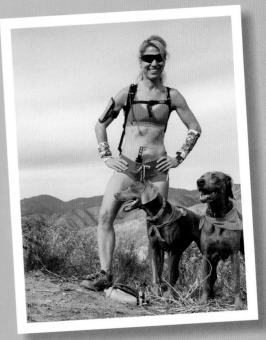

In canine conditioning, much of our strength exercises are targeted to strengthen the dog's core muscles (abdominals, obliques, and back muscles). Core strengthening is the single most beneficial training we can build in a dog, as it supports the dog's frame.

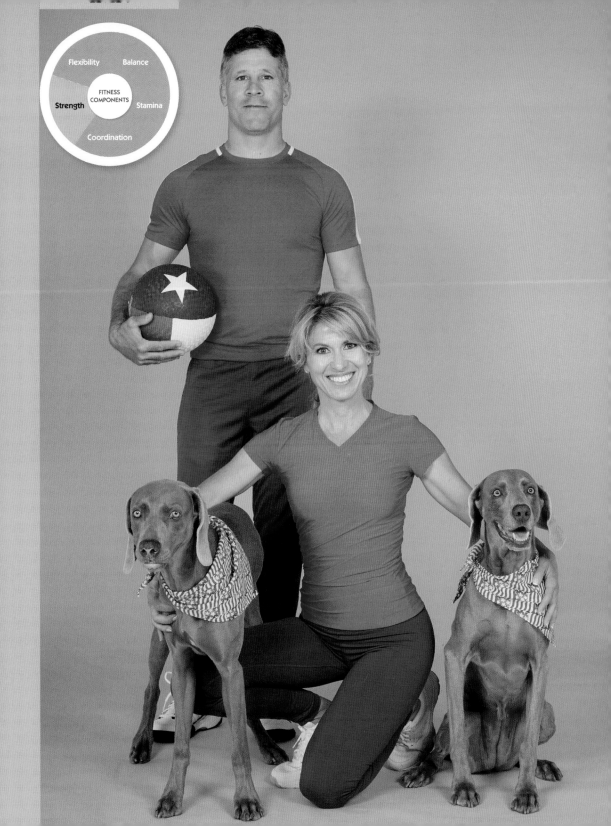

FITNESS COMPONENTS

Flexibility   Balance

Strength   Stamina

Coordination

Crawl Tunnel

TECHNIQUE: MOLDING

BENEFIT: STRENGTHEN CORE/FRONT AND HIND LIMBS/HIP FLEXOR (ILIOPSOAS)

A dog's **core** is his abdominal muscles, obliques, and back muscles. A dog uses his core muscles in almost everything he does. His core is a stabilizer that supports erect posture. Core muscles protect the dog's spine. A weak core results in poor posture, which causes problems with his back, shoulders, neck, hips, and knees. This crawl-tunnel exercise strengthens your dog's core, and all four of his limbs as he crawls below a low ceiling.

Molding is the technique of using a prop to elicit the behavior. You can make a crawl tunnel with a series of chairs.

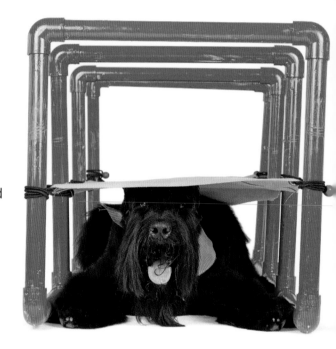

5 BENEFITS OF CORE STRENGTHENING

- Protects the back, making it less susceptible to injury
- Increases stability, decreasing stress to weaker limbs
- Strengthens the center of gravity, improving balance
- Improves posture
- Improves performance during exercise and sports

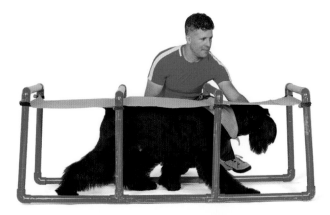

1 Use a toy or treat to lure your dog through a high tunnel.

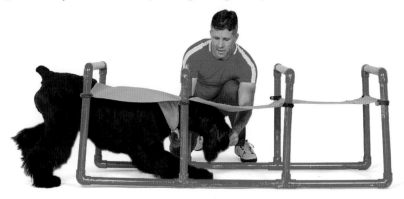

2 Slightly lower the ceiling and try again. Your dog will be more willing to crawl on a soft surface such as grass or carpet.

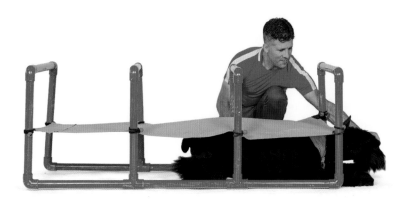

3 With a very low ceiling your dog will have to belly crawl. At this height, you may have to keep a lure in front of his nose the whole time.

Bar Jump

TECHNIQUE: EXPLOSIVE POWER

BENEFIT: STRENGTHENS HIND LIMBS

Explosive strength is producing a maximal amount of force in a minimal amount of time, such as jumping over a bar jump. The focus is on the speed of movement.

Rear limb muscles increase dogs' speed and power as well as helping them jump and extend their rear limbs. A strong rear helps a dog get up after laying down, helps him go up stairs, jump, and run. Rear limb muscles are usually the first muscles to atrophy as a dog ages, so it is important to keep up with hind-end exercises throughout the dog's lifetime.

HIND-END STRENGTH
The hind end consists of the muscles of the hips, knees, lower back (lumbar), and Achilles tendon. The hind end is responsible for power and strength.

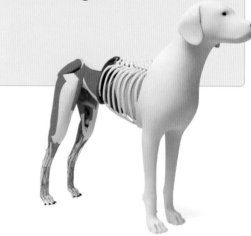

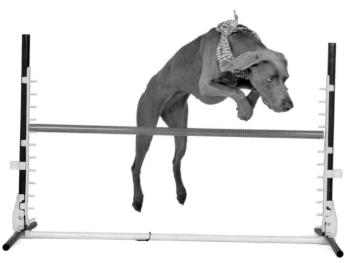

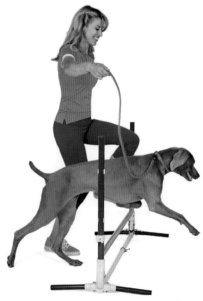

1 Set a bar jump at a low height. Get a running start to build enthusiasm, and run over the bar with your dog.

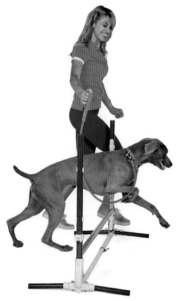

2 Next, run to the side and body pressure your dog toward the jump. If you use a leash, it should be slack.

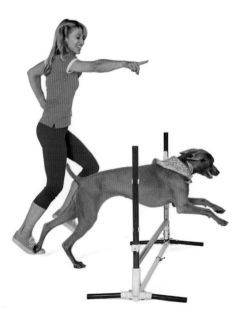

3 Instead of a leash, pretend you are holding an invisible leash, and launch your dog where you want her to go.

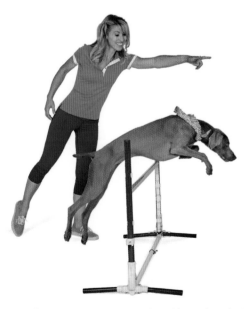

4 Gradually raise the bar. Use a bar that will fall off if your dog knocks it. Have good traction on the ground to avoid slipping.

Hoop Jump

TECHNIQUE:	EXPLOSIVE POWER
BENEFIT:	STRENGTHENS FRONT AND HIND LIMBS

Your dog's **front end** consists of the muscles of her neck, shoulders, and front legs.

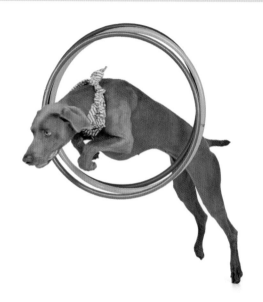

Front limbs are primarily responsible for weight bearing and stability. They are used to turn, land, and slow down or stop after movement. Dogs place the majority of their weight on their front legs. By strengthening our dog's front end stabilizer muscles, we improve her stability when running, landing, and walking on unstable surfaces.

The hoop-jump exercise works your dog's hind end during takeoff, and her front end when landing.

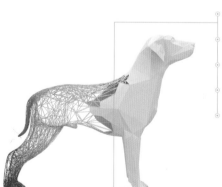

FRONT-END STRENGTH

- Stability while standing or climbing
- Reduced risk of injury when landing
- Improved balance on unstable surfaces
- Agility to make quick turns while running
- Ability to make sudden stops when running

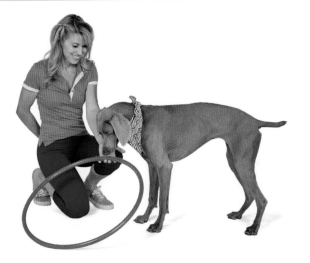

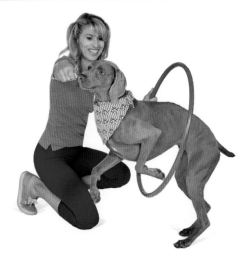

1. Introduce your dog to the hoop. Dogs may be apprehensive of it at first, especially if it has noisy beads inside.

2. Hold the hoop with the hand closest to the dog. With your other hand, use a treat to lure her through. You may have to hold the hoop all the way on the ground the first few times.

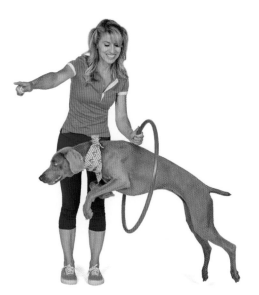

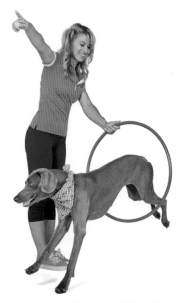

3. Hold the hoop higher. Use your pointed finger and a motivating "hup!" to encourage a big jump. A treat reward will help.

4. Landing holds some risk of injury. Jump only on surfaces with good traction (like grass) and keep your dog jumping straight.

Wall Stand

TECHNIQUE:	EXPLOSIVE POWER
BENEFIT:	STRENGTHENS LOWER BACK/INCREASES HIP FLEXOR (ILIOPSOAS) FLEXIBILITY

The wall-stand exercise builds core strength in your dog. Your dog will use **explosive power** to lift his front end, in one fell swoop, from the ground to an upright position.

There will be considerable variation in dogs' ability to perform this exercise based on their breed, weight, length of back, and age. A Chihuahua, for example, will require a lot less effort to wall stand than a Rottweiler.

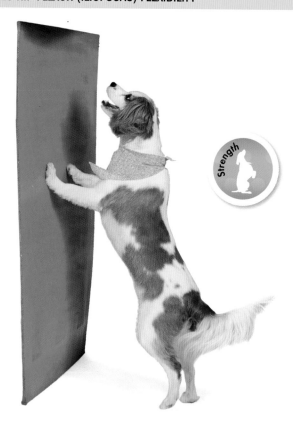

Strength

LONG-BACKED DOGS
Long-backed dogs, such as dachshunds and corgis, are more prone to disc herniation, which can lead to problems ranging from minor back pain to paralysis. These dogs will especially benefit from lower back exercises to help prevent back injury.

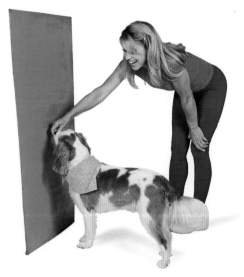

① Get your dog's interest with a treat held at his nose height, against the wall.

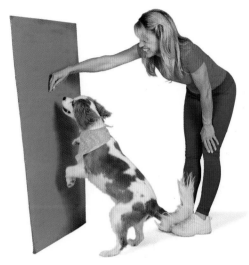

② Slide the treat up the wall, just out of his reach. If he doesn't attempt to go after it, coax him by sliding it back down and up again.

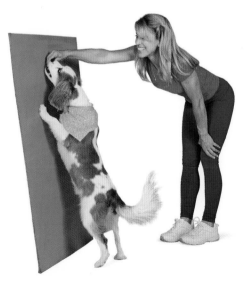

③ When your dog is in the correct position (up against the wall), hold him there 3 seconds by letting him nibble the treat.

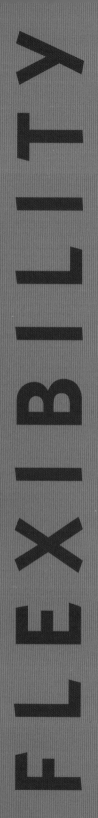

FLEXIBILITY

In level 1, we did **static stretches**; where we manually stretched the dog's limb and held the end position.

Dynamic stretching is a movement stretch where the dog will perform slow, controlled movements through full range of motion. Unlike static stretching, in dynamic stretching the dog does not hold an end position; the dog is always moving, or dynamic. Dynamic stretching warms the muscles and encourages blood flow to the area. Dynamic stretching is not the best for improving flexibility, but it is a good way to warm up for your sport and has been shown to improve performance.

Before or after stretching, your dog will benefit from **therapeutic massage,** which increases joint mobility and flexibility, helps break up scar tissue, enhances healing, and reduces stress.

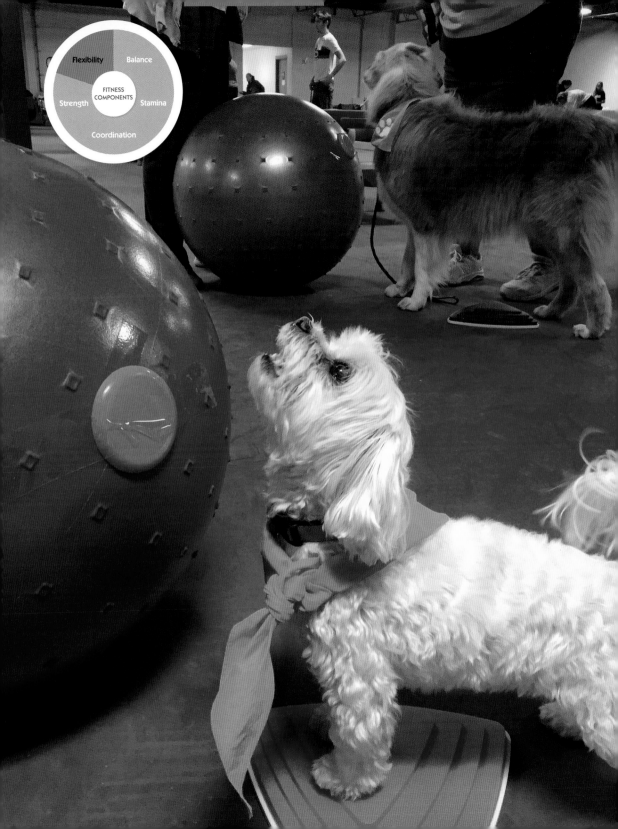

FITNESS COMPONENTS

Flexibility

Balance

Strength

Stamina

Coordination

Dynamic Stretch: Neck, Lying

TECHNIQUE:	DYNAMIC STRETCH/ROTATION STRETCH
BENEFITS:	IMPROVES NECK FLEXIBILITY

Dogs move their necks frequently to navigate through the world. A dog's neck muscles are quite small and, thus, get tight from all the strain. Decreased flexibility can limit a dog's ability to look up towards its owner or do well in sports. Stretching the muscles of the neck can increase flexibility to allow for full range of motion.

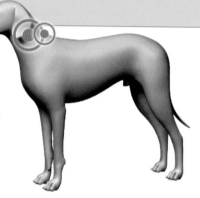

TARGET: Neck, cervical and spine muscles

REPEAT: 5 times on each side

With **dynamic stretching** we facilitate the dog moving her neck through its full range of motion, in a continuous, fluid motion. This stretches and warms the muscles and encourages blood flow, preparing the dog's body for exercise.

Begin with a small range of motion, and slowly increase the range.

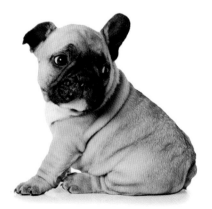

SHORT-NECKED DOGS will have a smaller range of motion in this exercise.

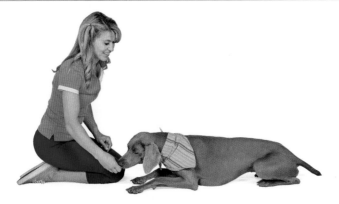

1 Start with your dog lying down. Hold a treat to her nose. She need not be in a Sphinx position, as in this photo, but may be askew on one hip.

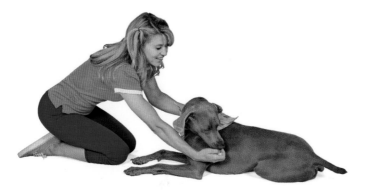

2 Move the treat from her nose to her shoulder blade. Hold the treat low, near her chest. Use your other hand to stabilize her neck, and feel the muscles.

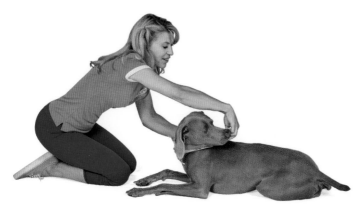

3 Raise the treat to her backbone. Notice how this stretches different muscles. Notice if your dog is more flexible on one side than the other.

Dynamic Stretch: Neck and Spine

TECHNIQUE:	DYNAMIC STRETCHING
BENEFIT:	IMPROVES NECK AND SPINE FLEXIBILITY

Increasing flexibility through stretching is one of the basic tenets of physical fitness. Athletes commonly stretch before and after exercise to reduce risk of injury and increase performance.

Build regular neck stretching into your dog's exercise regimen. Keeping her neck flexible will go a long way toward maintaining your dog's health, plus it takes only a few minutes to do.

The neck moves in four directions, so your stretching should be in those four directions. Different breeds will have more or less neck mobility, and short-necked dogs (such as bulldogs) may not be able to get their head between their paws.

TARGET: Spine, neck, and shoulder muscles.

REPEAT: 2–3 times on each side

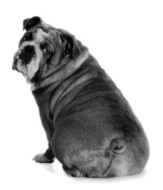

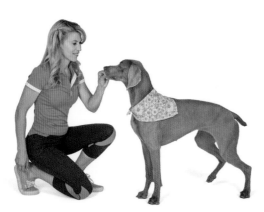

DOWN

1. Have the dog stand squarely. Hold a treat to her nose.

2. Lure the dog's head down between her feet. Keep the spine straight. Let her nibble the treat as long as you can.

UP

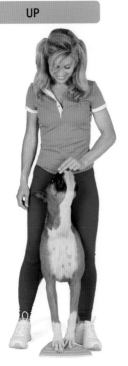

RIGHT   **LEFT**

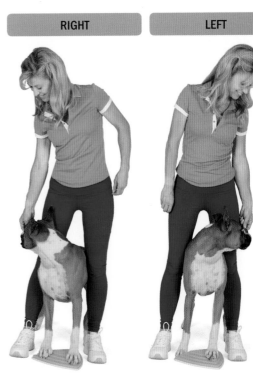

1. Use a treat to lure your dog to stretch his head up. Let him nibble or lick the treat to keep him in that position.

2. Gently clamp him with your legs. Move the treat to the left and the right to get a lateral neck stretch.

Dynamic Stretch: Shoulder Dip

TECHNIQUE: DYNAMIC STRETCH/EXTENSION

BENEFIT: IMPROVES SHOULDER FLEXIBILITY

Since the shoulder must move in many directions, flexibility is needed across all planes of movement.

Your dog's shoulders carry 60 percent of his weight, which puts a lot of stress on his shoulder and chest (pectoral) muscles. As a result, knots, muscles, and inflammation can occur. The shoulder dip stretch will stretch those tight muscles. This exercise should not be performed with dogs with elbow problems.

To get the most benefit from this stretch, start with a warm-up and end with a massage.

TARGET: Shoulder and chest muscles

REPEAT: 7–10 times

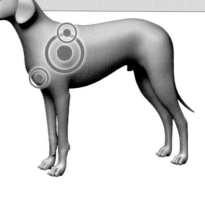

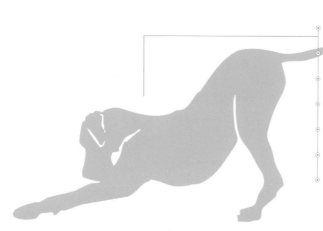

STRETCHING TIPS

- Warm up before stretching
- Strive for symmetry
- Focus on major muscle groups
- Don't bounce
- Hold the stretch
- Don't aim for pain
- Stretch routinely and consistently

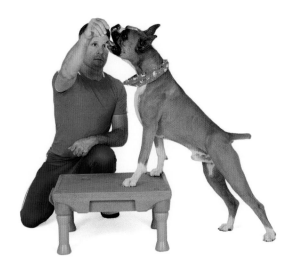

1. Use a treat to lure your dog to put his paws up on a platform (page 30).

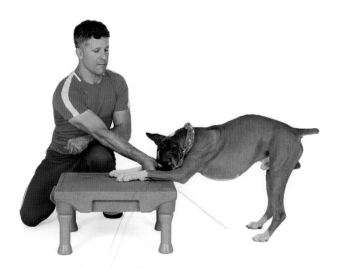

2. Slowly move the treat down to the edge of the platform. This should cause your dog to dip and extend his shoulders.

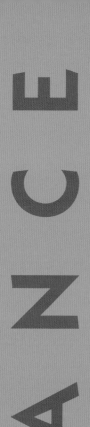

B A L A N C E

Over the last decade, there has been a shift from traditional methods of training to a variety of methods that are considered more functional or even more holistic in their nature.

Activities that include a balance or stability component have become commonplace. Instability training describes activities in which the dog is required to maintain control over his body position while he is interacting with an unstable surface under him.

Exercising on a surface that is unstable increases muscle activation, improves proprioception, betters neuromuscular control, and improves balance coordination.

In level 2, we will add more **Instability Training** exercises to our dog's training regime. Instability Training uses unstable surfaces to strengthen the core or trunk muscles.

Balance and stability activities enhance body awareness, encourage weight shifts and muscle contractions, and improve balance.

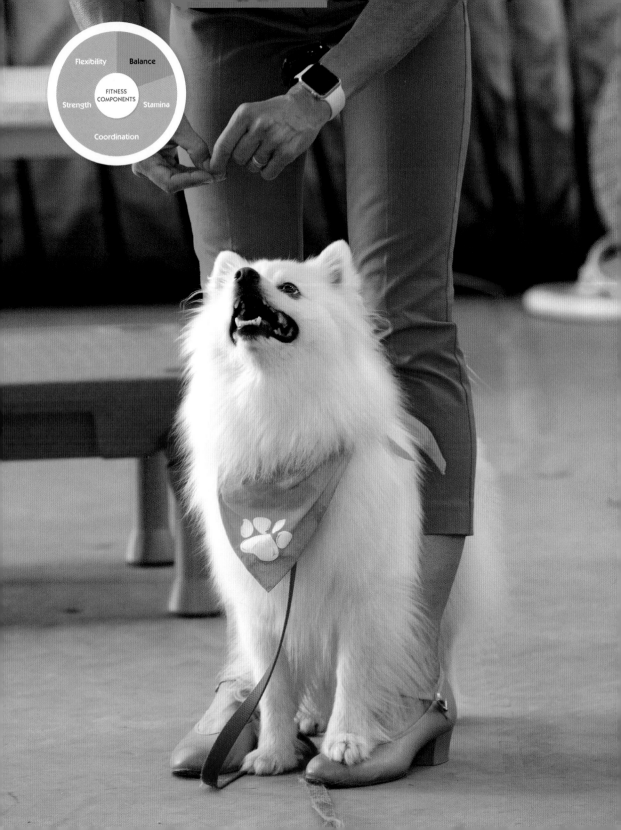

FITNESS
COMPONENTS

Flexibility   Balance

Strength   Stamina

Coordination

Paws up on Wobble Board

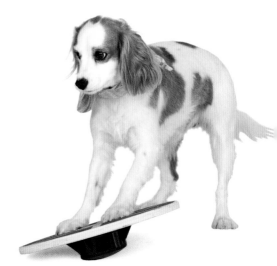

BALANCE

TECHNIQUE:	DYNAMIC BALANCE
BENEFITS:	IMPROVES BALANCE, REACTION TIME

A **wobble board** is an exercise device used to improve balance, functional strength, and mental focus. It will also strengthen the dog's lower leg muscles, which stabilize his wrists and ankles.

Wobble boards come in different shapes and sizes, but are basically a board with a small, often domed, piece on the bottom. When the dog steps on the wobble, it tilts, creating an unstable surface for him to balance upon. A lower dome produces smaller wobbles than a tall dome.

Wobble board training develops fast reflexes and quick reaction time for athletic training, as the dog must recover quickly from unpredictable tilts.

Wobble boards are commonly used for physical therapy.

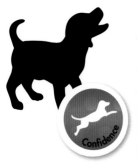

Confidence

GREAT FOR PUPPIES!
A wobble board is one of the first canine conditioning exercises introduced to puppies.

Fast reflexes aid sport performance and reduce injuries as the dog can recover quicker from loss of balance.

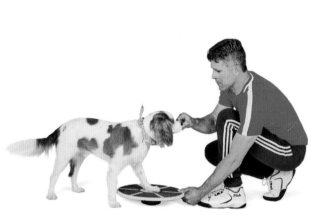

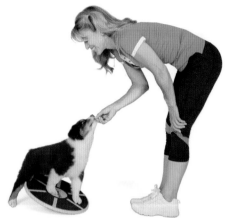

1 Stick your toe under the wobble board, or hold it with your hand to reduce its wobble. Use a treat to lure your dog to step on it.

2 Move the treat around to get your dog to shift his weight.

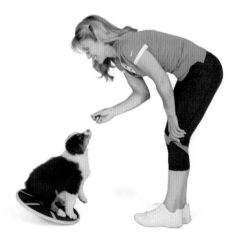

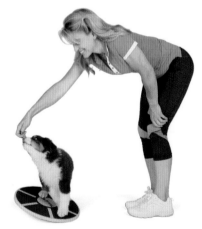

3 Continue to lure him forward to engage his back feet. There is no right or wrong way to wobble.

4 If your dog finds his balance, move the treat in different ways to get him to wobble.

Stand on a Peanut

BALANCE

TECHNIQUE: INSTABILITY TRAINING

BENEFIT: STRENGTHENS CORE AND FRONT AND REAR STABILIZER MUSCLES

The key to a well-functioning, injury-free body is balanced muscles; muscles on either side of the limb or trunk are equally developed.

When one muscle group overpowers the other (quadriceps are stronger than hamstrings, for example), this causes a cascading effect of compensation in the hips, knees, and shoulders.

When we train a dog on an unstable object, like an inflatable peanut, all of his muscles are engaged. The weak muscle will be the muscle that gets the greatest workout.

INSTABILITY TRAINING
When your dog stands on the peanut, it will start to vibrate; this is good! The vibration is giving the workout.

TIME: 5–30 seconds each repetition

REPEAT: Several times, for a total of 1–3 minutes

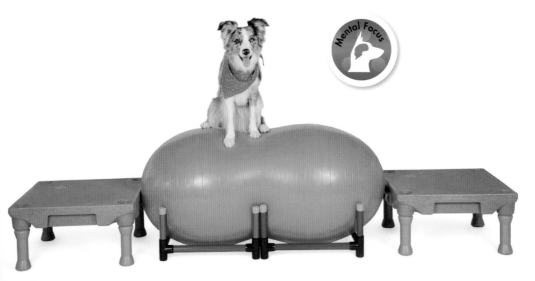

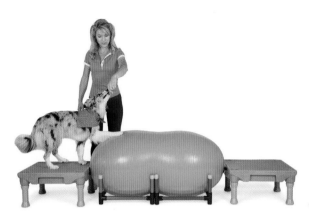

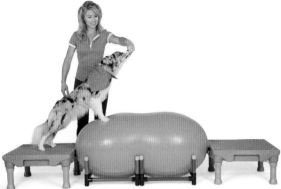

1. Secure the peanut in two Magic Squares. Set a platform at either end for safety. It's usually easiest to introduce your dog to the peanut by using a treat.

2. Let your dog make the decision on his own to step on the peanut, to avoid a traumatic episode. Just two feet is a good start.

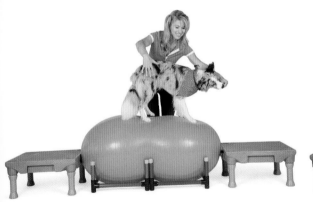

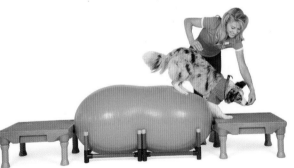

3. Dogs sometimes lose their balance and fall off the peanut. Always keep a hand guarding your dog.

4. Control the exit. Don't let your dog leap off the end. Use a treat low on the platform to slow him down and bring him off carefully.

Balance Beam

TECHNIQUE: LATERAL BALANCE

BENEFITS: IMPROVES BALANCE, PROPRIOCEPTION, AND REACTION TIME

This exercise is pretty straightforward, but it is accomplishing several things. It is honing your dog's **lateral balance** (side-to-side balance). It is also using your dog's peripheral vision and depth perception, which is needed for quick reaction time (yes, a dog can be trained to have faster reflexes!)

The balance beam exercise is also a confidence building challenge.

> **TIP!**
> Does your dog jump off the side? Place the balance beam alongside a wall. Body block him from the other side.

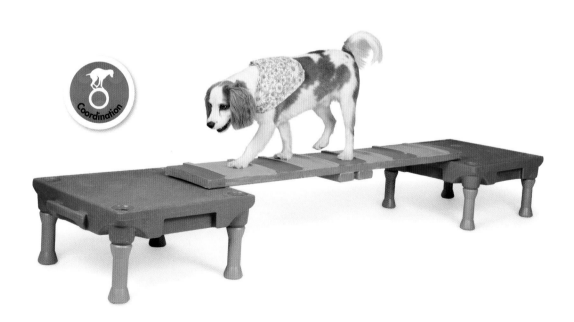

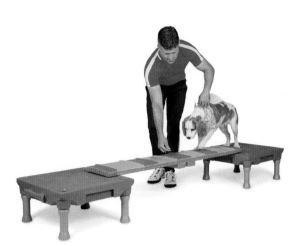

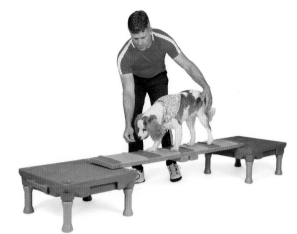

1. Erect a beam with a sturdy entrance and exit platform. Hold a treat low, next to the board (so your dog can see his feet as well as the board).

2. Keep luring him with treats. Use your other hand to guard his body in case he starts to fall, or decides to jump.

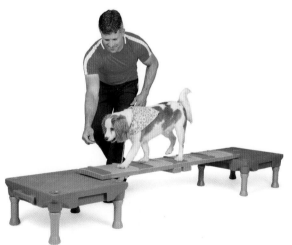

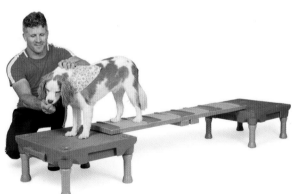

3. Have several treats in your hand. Give them to your dog along the way, or set them in a line along the beam.

4. Control the exit. Dogs tend to take a leap onto the platform, which is not a great idea. Slow your dog down with your voice or hand.

STAMINA

There are two types of Stamina.

Cardiovascular stamina (often called cardio) is the ability of the heart, lungs, and blood circulation to provide enough oxygen to working muscles. This type of conditioning is experienced in exercises such as running on the treadmill, learned in
level 1.

Muscle stamina is the second type of stamina. Muscle stamina is the ability of muscles to function for the length of the physical activity.

Training for Muscle Endurance:
Resistance training with moderate to low weights and high repetitions is the most effective method to improve muscular endurance and high-intensity (or strength) endurance. In level 2, we will use resistance training to build the dog's muscle stamina.

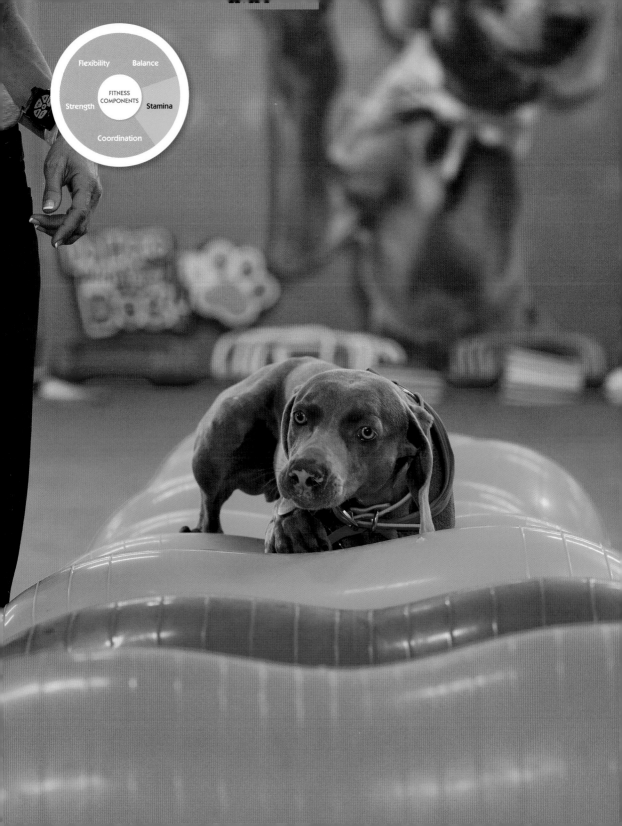

FITNESS COMPONENTS

Flexibility Balance

Strength Stamina

Coordination

Weight Pull

TECHNIQUE:	RESISTANCE TRAINING/HIGH-INTENSITY INTERVAL TRAINING (HIIT)
BENEFIT:	OVERALL MUSCLE STRENGTH AND STAMINA

In this exercise, the dog does **resistance training** (weight training) by pulling a tire. There are several ways to do this exercise.

CARDIO:
Have your dog pull a low weight for a longer time.

MUSCLE STAMINA:
Have your dog pull a heavy weight, focusing on muscle strength rather than cardio.

HIGH-INTENSITY INTERVAL TRAINING (HIIT):
Three all-out 30-second bursts of intense effort, with 1 minute of recovery time between each, has been shown in humans to be as beneficial for cardiovascular health as a 30-minute jog.

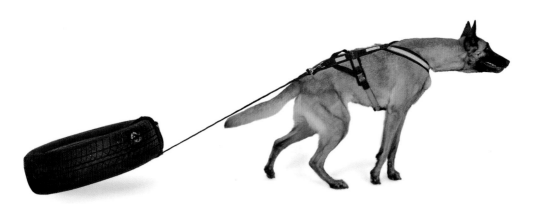

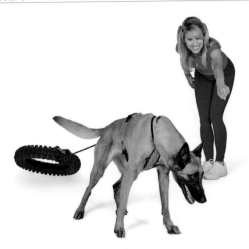

1 Outfit your dog in a well-fitting pulling harness, such as one used for dog mushing. It will have padding and a ring on the back, near the dog's hind end, to distribute the weight. Attach a lightweight tire, and let your dog pull it a short way to his food bowl.

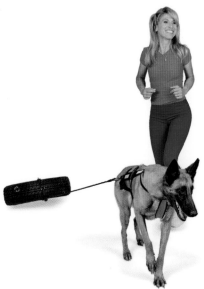

2 As your dog improves, you can increase the weight to a bigger tire. Many dogs will no longer need a food reward, but will be motivated to run alongside you.

COORDINATION

A lot of our dog's coordination relies on his **vision**. Drills can improve his central and peripheral vision, as well as his ability to react quickly and accurately. This will strengthen neuromuscular pathways between his eyes, his brain, and his reflexes, which will improve his reaction time.

To improve central vision, practice tossing a tennis ball or treat to your dog, which will boost eye-mouth coordination. Improve peripheral vision by tossing the ball or treat overhead or slightly to the left or right of your dog. He may miss a lot, at first, but as his brain adapts, he'll get faster.

In this chapter, your dog will learn to touch a target stick with his nose. This useful drill will improve your dog's eye-nose coordination.

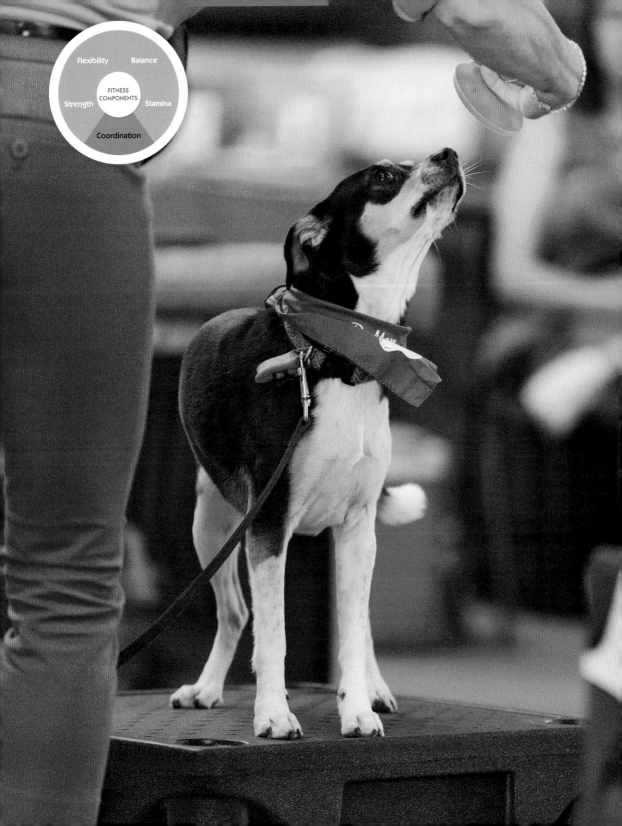

FITNESS COMPONENTS

Flexibility

Balance

Strength

Stamina

Coordination

Targeting: Touch Pad

TECHNIQUE: TARGETING

BENEFITS: FOUNDATION SKILL TO BE USED TO POSITION YOUR DOG

In previous exercises, our dog learned to nose-touch a target (our hand, a disc, or a target stick). It this exercise our dog will learn to target with his feet.

A **touch pad** is useful not only as a way to send your dog to a spot, but it will be a useful canine conditioning tool when we do 2-on/2–off exercises where we want our dog to place his front feet on a mark.

A good touch pad will have traction and a few inches (5 cm) of height to it.

TARGETING

- Nose touch your hand

- Nose touch a disc

- Foot touch a touch pad

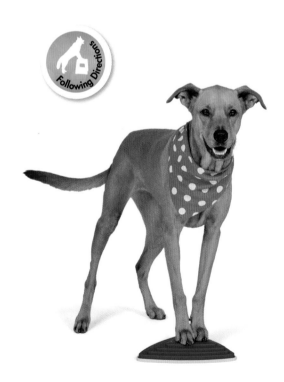

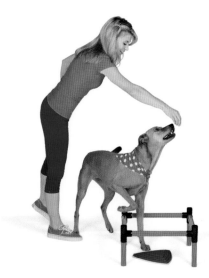

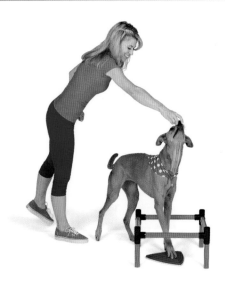

1 Your dog will have an easier time learning the touch-pad concept if the touch pad is on something or in something, such as a Magic Square.

2 Tell your dog "target!" and coax him in. Give him a treat when he is on the touch pad.

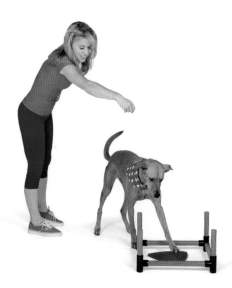

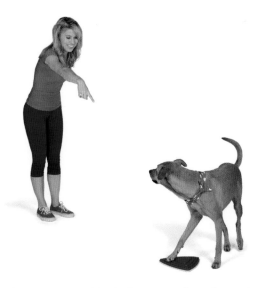

3 Turn the Magic Square upside down to make it lower. Try it again and coax your dog in.

4 Remove the Magic Square, and send your dog to the touch pad. Always give a treat while your dog is in the correct position, on the touch pad, and not after he has gotten off.

Cavalettis

COORDINATION

TECHNIQUE:	STRIDE REGULATION/RHYTHMIC MOVEMENT TRAINING
BENEFIT:	IMPROVES RHYTHM/IMPROVES PROPRIOCEPTION

Cavalettis are a series of small, regularly spaced hurdles used to improve a dog's balance, to adjust his length of stride, and to loosen and strengthen his muscles. They build a dog's confidence and improve his proprioception as he learns to stretch, lift, and use all four legs in a more deliberate manner.

Cavalettis are often used in sets of six, placed in a row, but have nearly unlimited ways they can be configured. Used at a low height, they encourage a proper length of stride. By being set closer or farther apart than a dog's natural stride, they encourage lengthening or shortening of the stride.

Set at higher settings, they become small jumps to introduce young dogs to jumping.

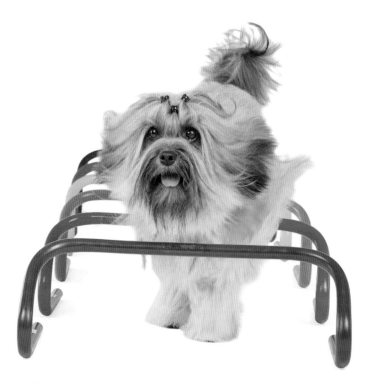

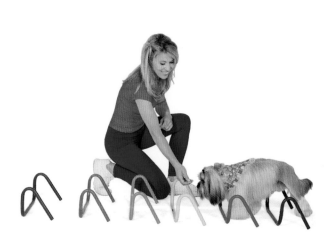

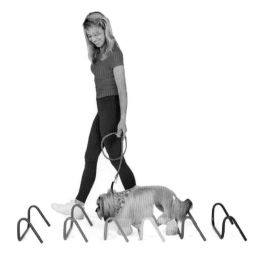

1 Set the cavalettis low to the ground, and equally spaced. Use a treat to lure him through. Hold the treat low to the ground, so he can see his feet as well as the treat.

2 After the first few times, use a leash instead of a treat, as treats are distracting for the dog.

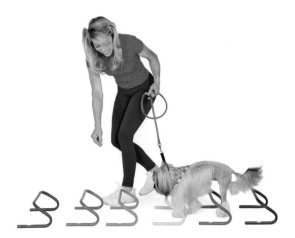

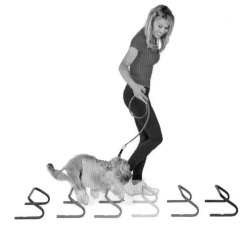

3 Set the cavalettis higher. You do not need to teach the dog how to go through the cavalettis; simply walk him through a number of times and he will improve on his own.

4 Experiment with different spacing, and notice how it changes your dog's stride. As with all exercises, do them in both directions.

Tight Circle

TECHNIQUE:	TARGETING
BENEFIT:	IMPROVES FOOT-PLACEMENT, PROPRIOCEPTION, AND BALANCE

Balance and proprioception go hand in hand. Good balance keeps your dog's weight evenly distributed, and good proprioception keeps her from tripping over her own feet. Balance is easiest when the four feet are in a wide stance. It becomes significantly more difficult when all four feet are positioned in a small spot.

Proprioception loss in dogs can lead to dragging of the foot when trying to walk, tripping, decreased coordination, or improperly placing the foot down when stepping. These may be signs of neurological issues and should be evaluated by a veterinarian. Proprioception is usually diminished after surgery (such as cruciate surgery) because the dog is not putting the injured leg down on the ground normally, or after a back injury or chronic disease such as Degenerative Myelopathy.

Activities that challenge your dog's balance are important for retraining proprioception. Affected limbs will not only grow stronger as weight is placed onto them, but the dog will also learn to sense the type of surface their foot is standing on. In this exercise, we work on a dog's coordination by having her spin in a tight circle, deliberately lifting and placing each foot. It is often the case that a dog is better at circling in one direction than the other, so train both.

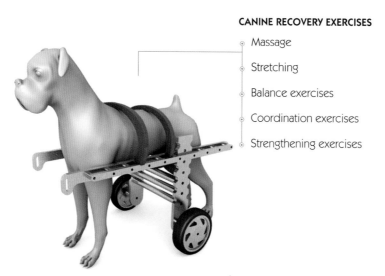

CANINE RECOVERY EXERCISES

Massage

Stretching

Balance exercises

Coordination exercises

Strengthening exercises

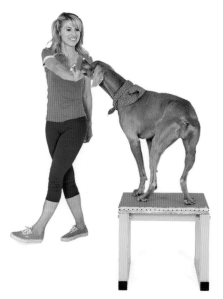

1 Set your dog on a small platform. Hold a treat or target disc at her nose height.

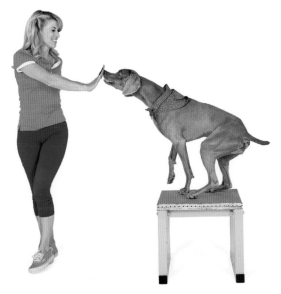

2 Walk around the platform, encouraging her to spin a circle to follow your hand.

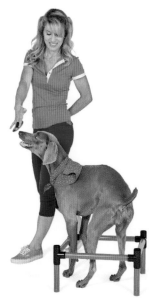

3 Alternately, try the same exercise with your dog's feet confined in a Magic Square.

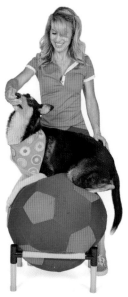

4 Combine elements and try to have your dog circle on top of a fit ball.

Rainbow Ladder: Front Paws Only

COORDINATION

TECHNIQUE: LATERAL MOVEMENT

BENEFIT: IMPROVE PROPRIOCEPTION/FRONT-END AWARENESS

In level 1, your dog learned to maneuver through the rungs of a ladder, walking forward. In this exercise, your dog will side-step his front feet through the rungs. Sidestepping, or **lateral movement**, is not a common natural behavior for a dog, and is one that can be improved through practice.

REPEAT: 3–4 times on each side

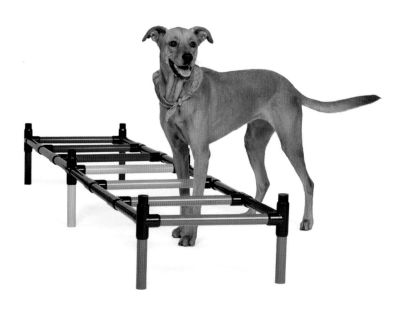

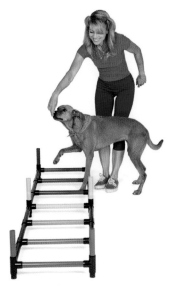

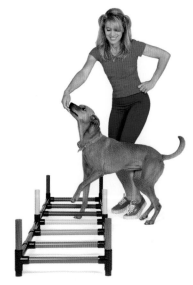

1. Set your ladder at a low height. Use a treat to lure your dog to step into the squares with both of his front feet.

2. Keep his head centered over the rungs by letting him nibble the treat. Use your leg to body-pressure his hind end sideways.

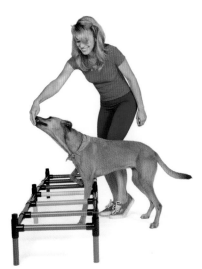

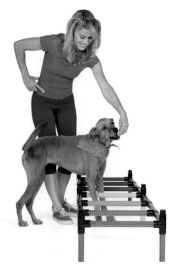

3. Raise the ladder height. Hold the treat so that his head is slightly leading his back end; we don't want him leading with his rear.

4. Practice in both directions; sidestep left, and sidestep right.

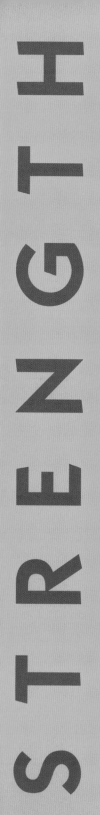

In level 1, we learned about the importance of core strengthening for our dog; as a weak core can cause a cascading effect of problems with the dog's hips, knees, shoulders, and neck.

In level 1, we also practiced hind-end strengthening as used in jumping, and front-end strengthening, used to land, stop, and turn.

Level 2 introduces **neck-strengthening exercises** to build strength and stability. The neck is an often overlooked muscle group, but one that requires as much attention, if not more, as the other muscle groups.

Neck muscles move the dog's head through various ranges of motion— extension, forward flexion, lateral flexion, and rotation—that he uses on a daily basis. These muscles can be strengthened by performing resistance exercises. This will help them function more effectively and may prevent neck pain, or back injury which can be debilitating.

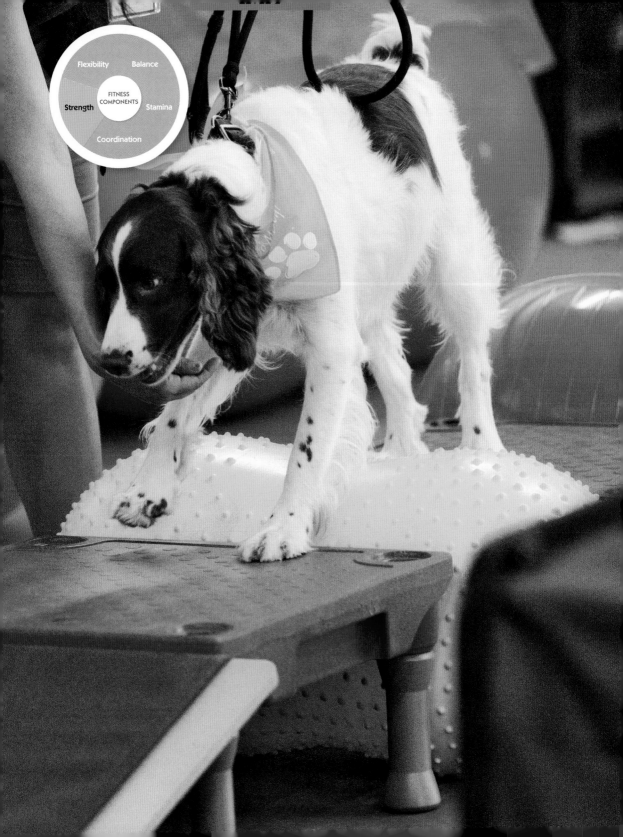

FITNESS
COMPONENTS

Flexibility   Balance

Strength   Stamina

Coordination

Neck: Push a Carpet Roll

TECHNIQUE: RESISTANCE TRAINING

BENEFIT: STRENGTHENS NECK EXTENSION MUSCLES

Neck strengthening is a beneficial, and often overlooked, part of your dog's conditioning plan. As a dog ages and weakens, he tends to let his head hang closer to the ground.

This exercise specifically targets those muscles used in holding the dog's head up: his trapezius muscle (at back of his neck) and his brachiocephalic muscle (at the sides of his neck). There are also many smaller neck muscles that will benefit from this exercise.

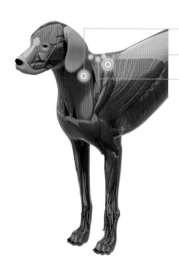

NECK STRENGTHENING

- Brachiocephalic muscle
- Trapezius muscle
- Many smaller muscles of the neck that stabilize the spine

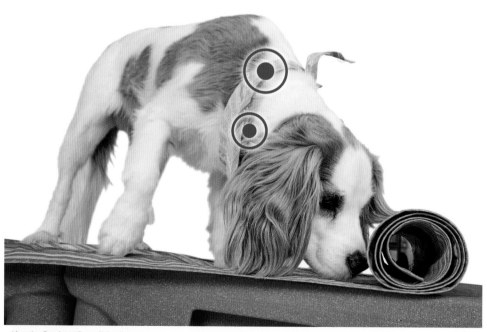

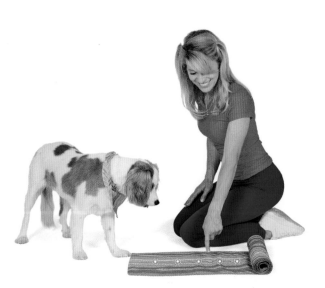

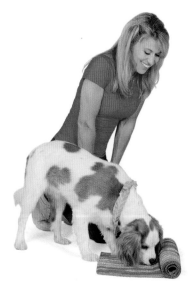

1. Use a table runner or hallway carpet runner. Lay a line of treats about 6 inches (15 cm) apart down the length of the runner. Let your dog watch as you roll it up.

2. Point out the first treat to him, and let him get it. As he nudges under the roll, the next treat will become exposed. If he loses interest, unroll and reroll the carpet to show him the treat.

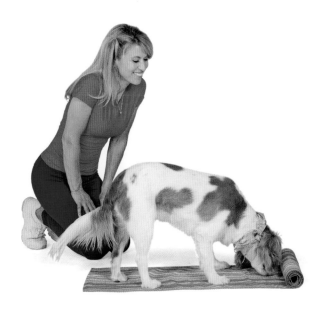

3. As your dog improves, you can phase out the line of treats and put just one dog biscuit at the very end.

Paws up on My Arm

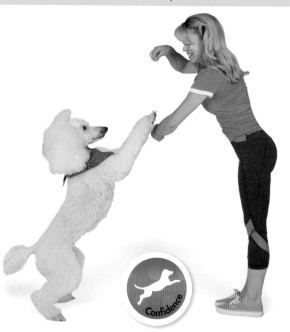

TECHNIQUE:	EXPLOSIVE POWER
BENEFIT:	STRENGTHENS CORE/BACK EXTENSION/THORACIC AND LUMBAR MUSCLES/HIND-END

A dog's thoracic and lumbar muscles (his **epaxial muscles**) are found on the two sides of his spine. This central portion of the vertebra column acts a bridge offering support for the two sets of his limbs. They also helps to protect his spine as well as providing an anchor for the other strong muscle groups of the dog's body.

In this exercise, we train the dog to use his back and rear leg muscles to lift his front paws onto our arm. Alternately, if the dog is unable to make that explosive power lift (perhaps he is older, overweight, or a giant or stout breed dog) lift his paws manually onto your arm and have him support himself in that position.

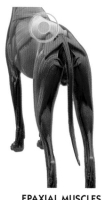

Confidence

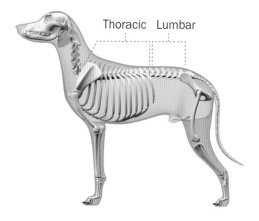

Thoracic   Lumbar

EPAXIAL MUSCLES

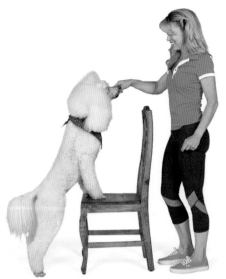

1 Your dog has already learned to put his paws up on a platform (page 30). Now have him put his paws up on a sturdy chair.

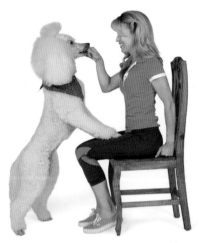

2 Sit in the chair, and have him put his paws up on your thighs.

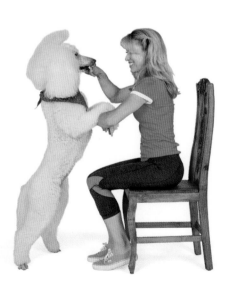

3 Lure him to put his paws on your arm. Stay seated in the chair, as your dog will feel more confident if your body is solid and stable.

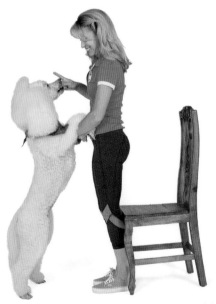

4 If your dog is tall enough, have him put his paws on your arm while you are standing.

Localized Landing Platform Jump

TECHNIQUE:	LOCALIZED LANDING
BENEFIT:	STRENGTHENS HIND END AND FORE LIMBS/TEACHES JUMP COLLECTION

When jumping, we want the dog to make an ideal arc and a straight, flat (not vertical) landing. This results in faster agility runs, fewer knocked bars, and fewer injuries. We can condition a dog to jump correctly by training localized landings.

With **localized landing**, we have the dog jump from platform to platform, thus forcing them to jump thoughtfully by making the landing an integral part of the plan. It teaches the dog **purposeful collection** in jumping. We use a hoop between platforms to get the desired height/arc of the jump.

Platform jumps use explosive strength, which utilizes your dog's hind-end as he leaps and his front end and shoulders as he lands.

> **LOCALIZED LANDING**
> Localized landing teaches your dog how to **collect**, **jump**, and **land**. There are three variables we can manipulate
>
> - Distance between platforms
> - Size of the landing platforms
> - Height of hoop

HIGH-ARC JUMP
When jumping over a bar jump

LONG, FLAT JUMP
When jumping far in dock diving

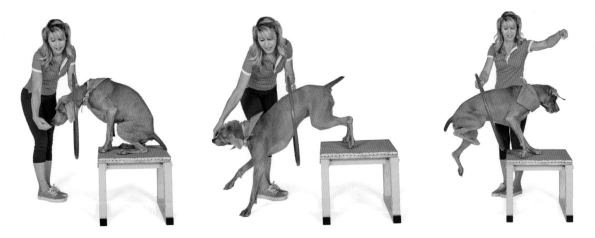

1. Use a treat to practice having your dog jump onto and off of a platform through a hoop.

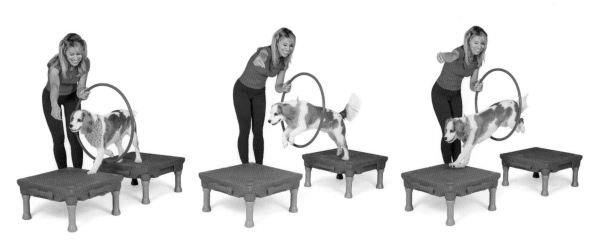

2. Start with a small separation between platforms. Hold the hoop in the hand closes to your dog, and lure him through. Gradually increase the distance between platforms and the height of the hoop.

Tug

TECHNIQUE:	RESISTANCE TRAINING
BENEFIT:	STRENGTHENS NECK AND CORE

Tugging on a rope or toy strengthens your dog's neck, back, and front and hind leg muscles. For the purpose of strength training, don't make this an aggressive game.

Think low and slow. Encourage just enough resistance to enable the muscles to stretch comfortably. The higher you hold the toy, relative to the dog's body, the more load will be placed on the dog's back legs. Conversely, the lower you hold the toy, the more load will be placed on her front legs.

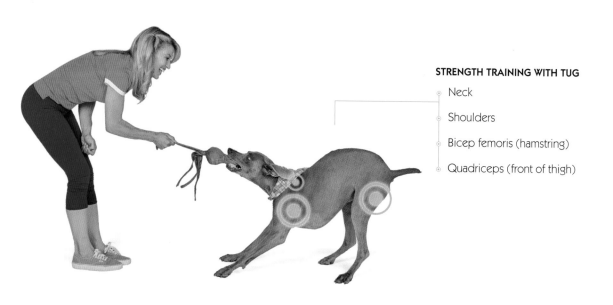

STRENGTH TRAINING WITH TUG

- Neck
- Shoulders
- Bicep femoris (hamstring)
- Quadriceps (front of thigh)

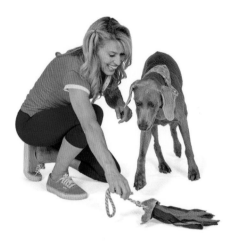

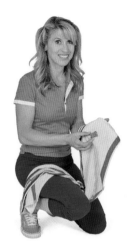

1. Encourage your dog's natural prey drive with a leather or fur toy that has fringes or squeakers. Make it skitter away from your dog like a real prey animal. When she catches it, tug slightly.

2. Some dogs are natural tuggers. If your dog is not, tie a treat in a knotted towel. Stick additional treats in the crevices of the knot.

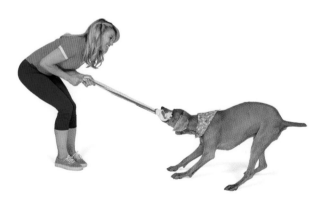

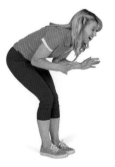

3. Encourage your dog to get the treats. Be playful and encouraging. Dogs are sometimes more willing to tug outdoors.

4. As soon as your dog tugs, let her pull the towel from your hand (the game is more fun if she wins!)

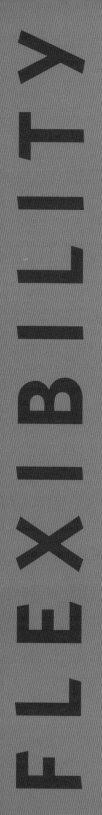

FLEXIBILITY

Focus on your dog's hips, shoulders and back, where stretching is especially beneficial.

Without **back flexibility**, back muscles become tight, resulting in reduced range of motion. When a dog goes past that reduced range, an injury can occur to the muscles, tendons, and ligaments. By improving a dog's back flexibility, we increase his range of motion and lower his risk of an injury.

A strong back that is also flexible allows your dog to twist, bend, and reach with greater ease and agility. A back-flexibility program should includes stretches for the back muscles, as well as the chest, abs, obliques, and hip flexors.

Benefits of back flexibility:

- Increased range of motion
- Injury prevention
- Improved circulation
- Better posture

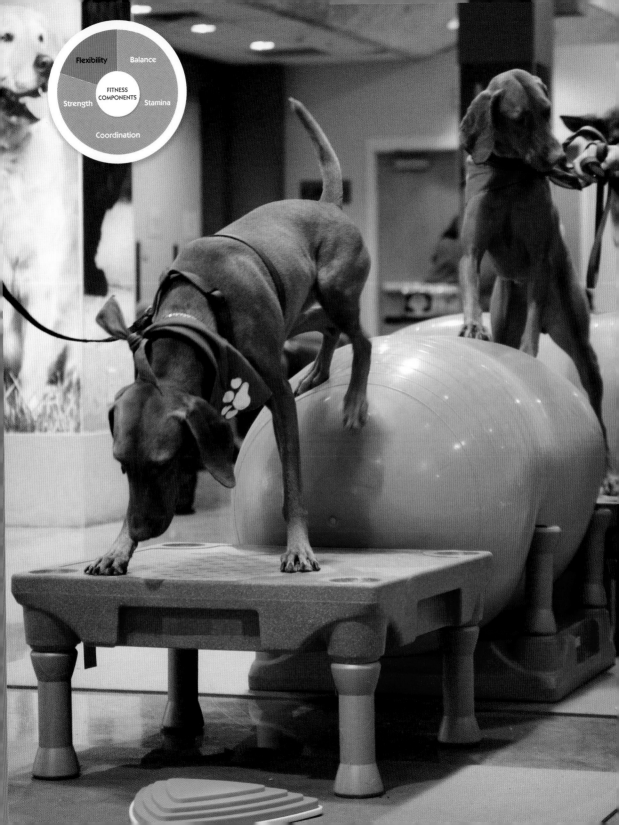

FITNESS
COMPONENTS

Flexibility

Balance

Strength

Stamina

Coordination

Dynamic Stretch: Spine

TECHNIQUE: DYNAMIC STRETCH/FLEXION

BENEFIT: IMPROVES SPINE, NECK, AND SHOULDER FLEXIBILITY

This dynamic stretch takes your dog through a full **range of motion** as she flexes her neck by curling her chin toward her chest. In the second stretch, we lure the dog to curve her head sideways, toward her shoulder.

Your dog has already trained on the **Shoulder Dip** exercise (page 66), so this exercise should be an easy transition.

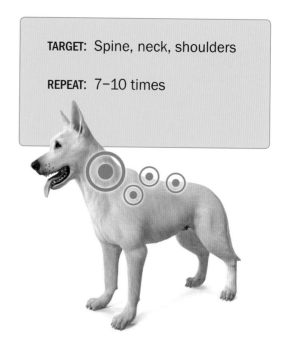

TARGET: Spine, neck, shoulders

REPEAT: 7–10 times

SPINE STRETCHING IMPROVES CIRCULATION
Tension in the spine muscles affects circulation. Stretching encourages circulation by helping blood move to the muscles and joints.

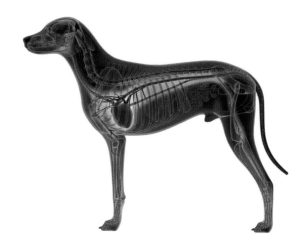

EXERCISE 1: CHIN TO CHEST

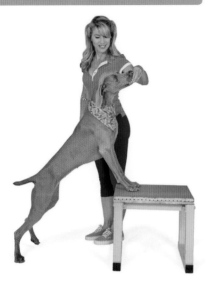

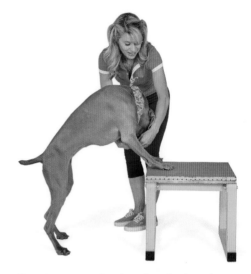

1 Hold a few small treats in each hand. Use one hand to lure your dog to put her paws on a platform.

2 Bring your other hand under her chest to join with the first hand.

EXERCISE 2: NOSE TO SHOULDER

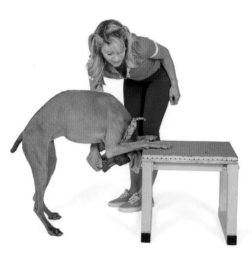

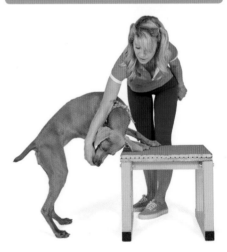

3 Remove your first hand and lure her chin as far as you can to her chest. Hold the stretch for 5 seconds.

4 Start again as in step 1, by luring her to place her front paws on the platform. Next, lure her nose as far as you can toward her shoulder. Hold the stretch for 5 seconds. Repeat with the opposite shoulder

Dynamic Stretch: Bow

TECHNIQUE:	**DYNAMIC STRETCH**
BENEFIT:	**IMPROVES FLEXIBILITY IN HIP FLEXORS, GROIN, SHOULDERS, LOWER BACK (LUMBAR SPINE) MUSCLES**

The **bow** is a natural stretch for dogs, and one they will often do when they first rise from a nap. This stretch specifically targets the hip flexors and lower back muscles. The hip flexors are muscles that enable your dog to move his legs and hips while walking, trotting, running, or jumping.

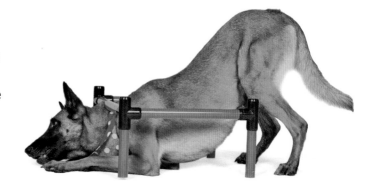

> **TARGET:** Hip flexors, shoulders, lower back muscles
>
> **REPEAT:** 7–10 times

3 BENEFITS THE BOW STRETCH

- Increased movement and flexibility in the hips and spine
- Improved conditioning of the lower back, hip, and leg muscles
- Reduction in arthritis-related discomfort and pain

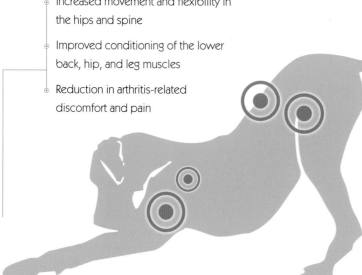

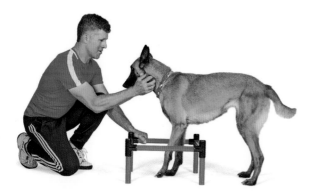

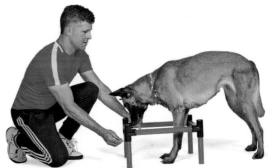

1. Use a treat to lure your dog to put his front paws inside a Magic Square. He should already be familiar with this request from the **touch pad** exercise (page 82).

2. While his front paws are in the Magic Square, show him a treat below the rung.

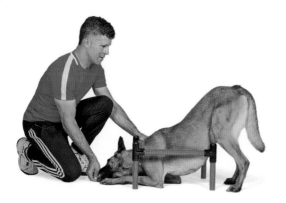

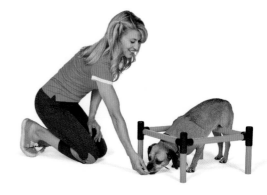

3. Your dog will go on his elbows to reach the treat. The back rung of the Magic Square will keep his rear up.

4. The same steps apply to little dogs.

Dogs who have suffered an injury, whether related to sports, surgery, or age, can benefit from balance training as part of their **rehabilitation** under veterinary guidance.

Canine physical therapists use balance training to aid in recovery by using it to strengthen and mobilize the injured muscles.

Pain can hinder a dog's natural awareness of his body's movements and will reduce his body movement. A dog is naturally less likely to move a joint freely when it is hurting. Consequently, reduced movement in the joint leads to reduced coordination and, therefore, leads to poor balance. Balance training utilizes the injured muscles and puts them through a range of motion, rehabilitating the injury.

Balance exercises are especially beneficial for senior dogs, whose proprioception becomes less effective as they age, putting them at greater risk of injury.

Balance exercises teach your dog's body to control the position of a deficient or an injured joint.

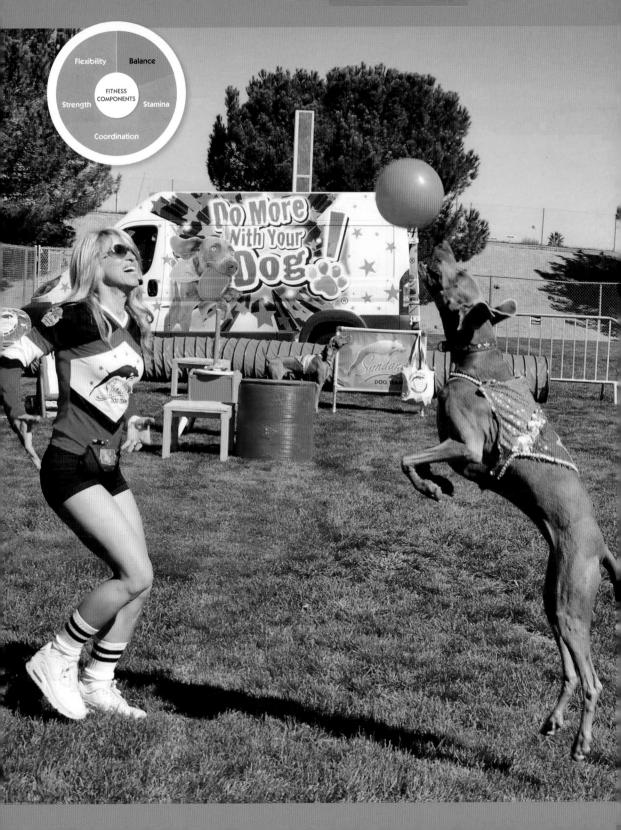

2-on/2-off Peanut

TECHNIQUE:	INSTABILITY TRAINING
BENEFIT:	IMPROVES BALANCE/STRENGTHENS SHOULDERS, BACK, AND HIP FLEXOR (ILIOPSOAS)

In level 2 your dog learned to stand on a peanut. This utilized **Instability Training** to tense and strengthen almost every muscle in your dog's body. By using Instability Resistance Training, we don't need to know which of our dog's muscles are weak; the weak muscle will automatically get the most strength training.

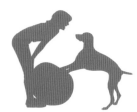

In this exercise, we will combine the **Touch Pad Targeting** skill (page 82) with the peanut to guide our dogs into a 2-on/2-off position.

This exercise will put a lot of weight on your dog's wrists, and should not be done if your dog has hyperextension (stretched ligaments) of these joints.

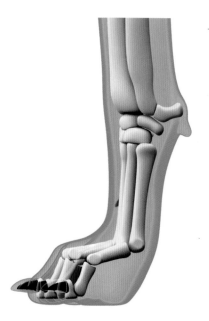

5 BENEFITS TO THE FOREFEET

- Increase bone density with weight-bearing exercise
- Strengthen stabilizer muscles
- Wrist extension for flexibility
- Toe extension for flexibility
- Improved paw-eye coordination to hit the touch pad

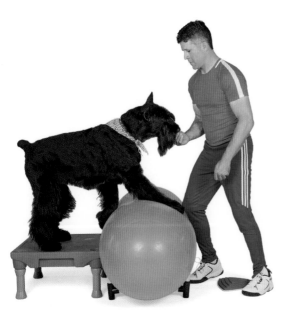

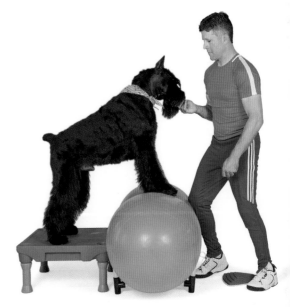

1 Stabilize the peanut in a Magic Square. Set a stable platform at one end and a touch pad at the other.

2 Lure your dog onto the peanut. Stabilize it with your knee.

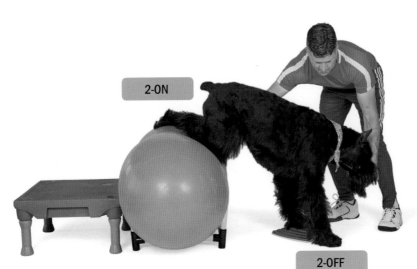

2-ON

2-OFF

3 Continue to lure your dog right over the other side by holding a treat over the touch pad. After a few seconds, have him walk forward off the peanut.

Stacking Pods

TECHNIQUE: DYNAMIC BALANCE

BENEFITS: ENCOURAGES SQUARE POSTURE/STRENGTHENS STABILIZER MUSCLES

Stacking pods are used to guide a dog to stand with correct, square posture—to improve her balance—and to target the muscles that enhance wrist and foot stability.

The muscles involved in balancing on stacking pods are those whose primary job is to stabilize joints in the limbs. This exercise strengthens the multiple forearm muscles that support the wrist and the lower hind leg muscles and Achilles tendon that support the hock (ankle).

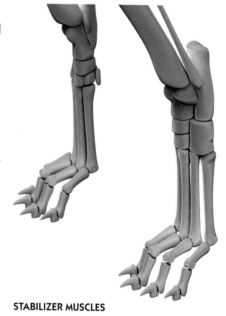

STABILIZER MUSCLES

- Stabilize joints in the limbs
- Support the wrist and lower hind leg muscles
- Support the Achilles tendon and ankle
- Aid in balance

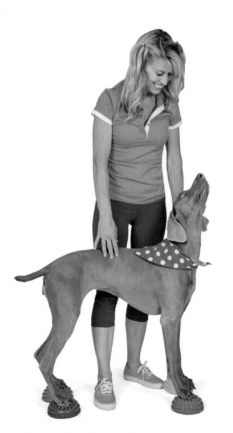

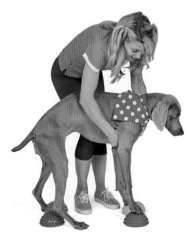

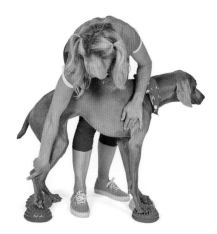

1. Set the pods so they line up with your dog's natural stance. Start with her front feet. Lift her chest and let her front feet lower until they are on top of the pods.

2. Manually place her back feet. Lift each by the hock (as dogs are squeamish about their feet) and place on a pod. It is normal for the dog to keep removing one or the other of her feet, at first.

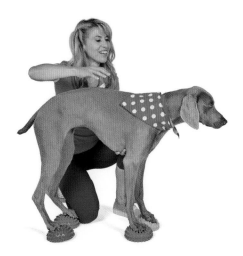

3. Once all four paws are situated, see if she can balance on her own for a few seconds. This will require tension in her wrists and ankles.

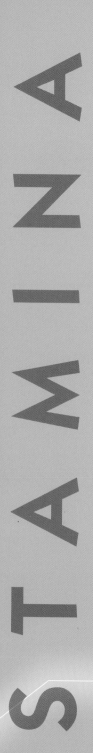
STAMINA

Physical therapy, under the guidance of a veterinarian, provides strengthening and stretching for dogs with dysfunction, injury, pain, or physical abnormalities. These techniques can make a significant difference in a dog quality of life.

The overall goal of veterinary **rehabilitation** is to restore, maintain, and promote optimal function and wellness, including

- Increased speed of recovery from injury or surgery
- Increased strength, endurance, and flexibility
- Improved performance and quality of movement
- Decreased possibility of injury recurrence through fitness

Conditions improved with physical therapy:

- Athletic conditioning
- Weight loss
- Muscle sprains/strains
- Wellness and injury prevention

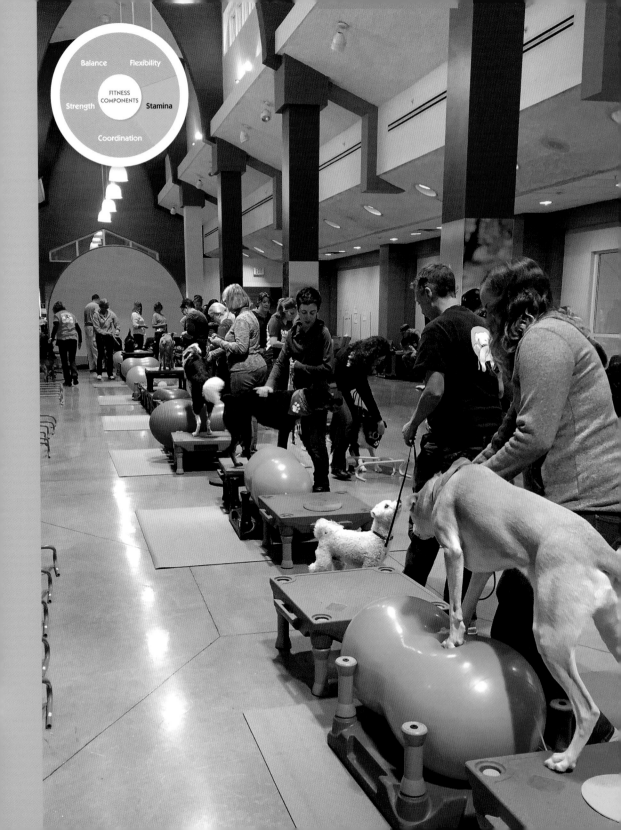

FITNESS COMPONENTS

Balance   Flexibility

Strength   Stamina

Coordination

Hydrotherapy

TECHNIQUE: LOW IMPACT EXERCISE

BENEFIT: IMPROVES MUSCLE STAMINA/RANGE OF MOTION/MUSCLE BUILDING/CARDIOVASCULAR

Hydrotherapy can be a dog walking on an underwater treadmill or assisted swimming. This low-impact exercise increases musculoskeletal and cardiovascular fitness. Hydrotherapy strengthens the dog's muscles while minimizing stress on his joints and bones through the buoyancy of the water. The warm water environment helps to increase overall flexibility and range of motion. Swimming is an incredible cardiovascular workout and is a wonderful way to increase your pet's strength or burn off some energy. Consult your veterinarian, however, as hydrotherapy can be dangerous for dogs with underlying or diagnosed heart and lung conditions.

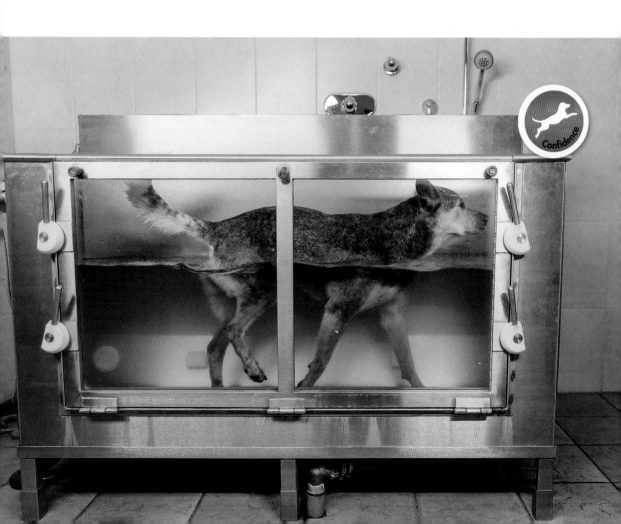

Confidence

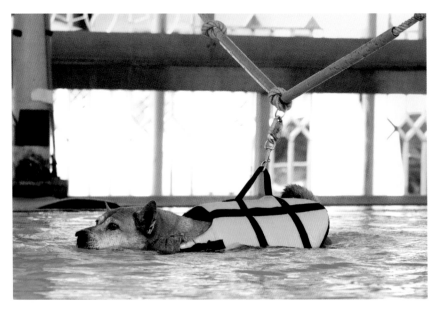

1 Life jackets and harnesses give a dog confidence in the pool and encourage full range of motion while swimming.

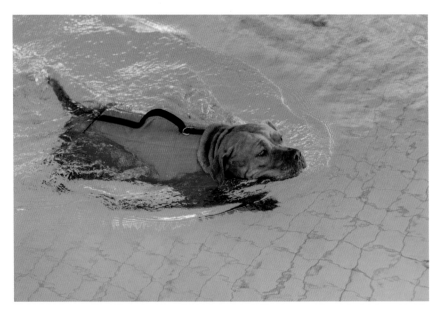

2 Low-impact, non weight-bearing exercises like swimming are used to rehabilitate an injury.

COORDINATION

Coordination is the dog's ability to synchronize and combine movements of various body parts at the same time. In levels 1 and 2, we trained **rhythmic movement** exercises where the dog repeated a specific movement over and over in a smooth coordinated motion (such as cavalettis and rainbow ladders).

Now, in level 3, we will introduce more **complex coordination** tasks, where the dog trots cavalettis that are in an arc (forcing him to stutter step on one side only), or rolling a barrel requiring him to walk forward with his hind legs and backward with his forelegs (much like rubbing your belly and patting your head at the same time!). Until the skill has been practiced and committed to muscle memory, it takes conscious effort to do the two conflicting actions, even though either one, individually, is very simple.

Learning coordinated movements helps **neural functioning**, making the dog's movements smarter and sharper.

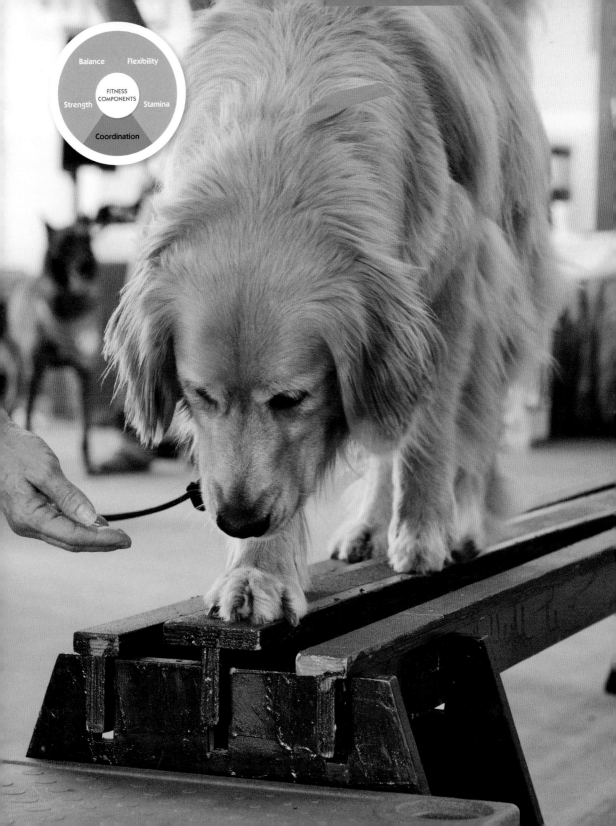

FITNESS COMPONENTS

Balance   Flexibility

Strength   Stamina

Coordination

Cavalettis: Irregular

TECHNIQUE: COMPLEX COORDINATION/ASYMMETRIC MOVEMENTS

BENEFIT: IMPROVES LIMB ISOLATION COORDINATION

In level 2, your dog trained on cavalettis and practiced trotting with all four feet in a rhythmical movement. In this exercise, we will set the cavalettis in specific patterns, which cause an **asymmetric gait**.

In a cavaletti arc, your dog may need to take a stutter step with his inside foot after every three hurdles. This unequal pattern will force your dog to consciously think about his foot placement.

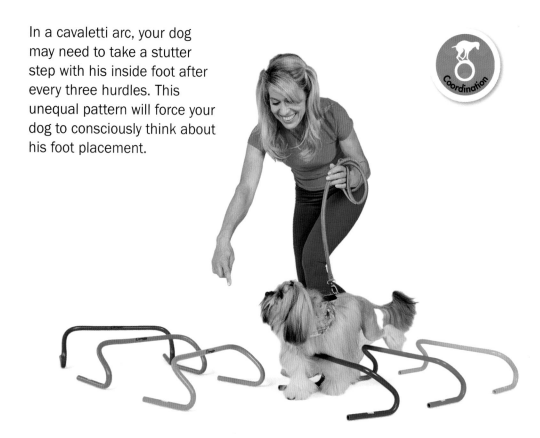

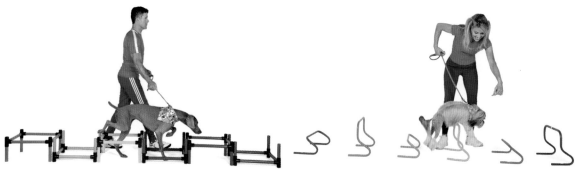

1 **High/low cavalettis walking:** walk your dog though a series of Magic Squares. It may take him a few walk-throughs to figure out a pattern.

2 **High/low cavalettis jumping:** set cavalettis equidistant apart. There needs to be enough space between them for your dog's four feet to land.

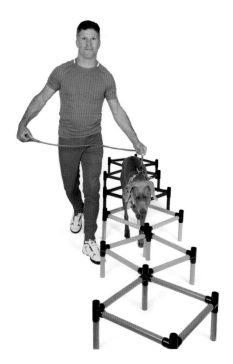

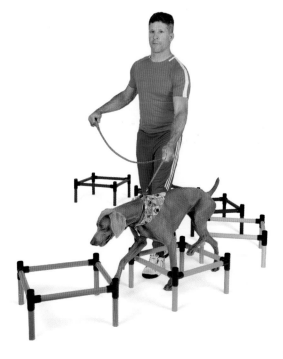

3 **Diamonds:** This complicated configuration of Magic Squares will perplex your dog. Walk through it slowly as he thinks about the placement of each individual foot.

4 **Arc:** With the Magic Squares in an arc, your dog will have to take more steps with one side of his body than with the other. Train in both directions.

Barrel Roll: 2 Feet

TECHNIQUE:	COMPLEX COORDINATION
BENEFIT:	IMPROVES FLEXIBILITY IN HIP FLEXORS (ILIOPSOAS), CORE, REAR AND FRONT LEG MUSCLES

The barrel roll exercise is deceptively complicated. By simply rolling the barrel (peanut) forward, your dog is walking forward with his hind legs, and walking backward with his forelegs. It's a little like rubbing your belly and patting your head at the same time! In addition to the complex coordination requirements, your dog will also be strengthening his core, hip flexors, shoulders, and forearms.

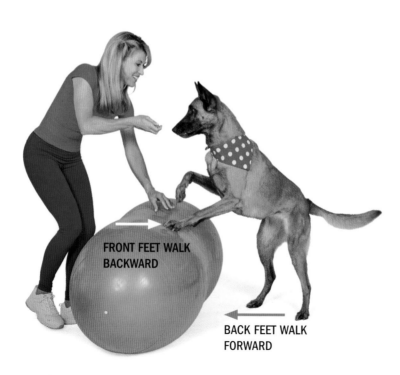

FRONT FEET WALK BACKWARD

BACK FEET WALK FORWARD

THE BARREL ROLLS FORWARD

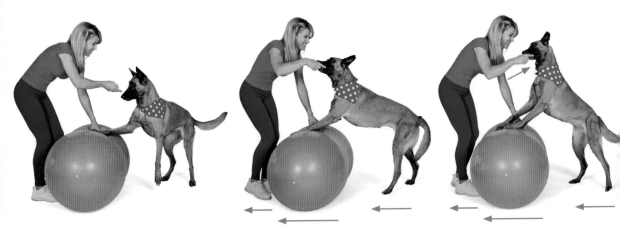

1 Stand on the opposite side of the barrel or peanut and stabilize it with your knees. Lure your dog to put her front paws up.

2 Take a step back and pull the peanut toward you. If your dog's elbows drop to the peanut, it is because you are pulling the treat too far in front of him. Instead, push your treat in toward his nose and up.

THE BARREL ROLLS BACKWARD

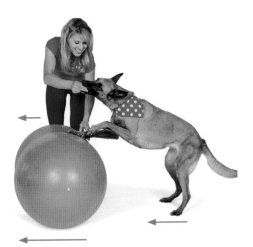

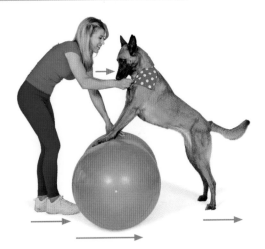

3 Another way to do this exercise is to stand alongside your dog and push the peanut forward with your hand.

4 Try it in the other direction; you walk forward and push the peanut toward your dog. This direction is more awkward. Make sure to keep the treat high and pushed in toward the dog.

Back-up Chute

TECHNIQUE: MOLDING

BENEFITS: BACK FEET COORDINATION

How often in a dog's daily life does she walk backward? Maybe once a week? Walking backward is a skill that benefits from practice. It is particularly challenging for the hind feet, as they must lift and reach and feel for the ground behind them.

There are different ways of teaching a dog to back up, but the chute method is quick, simple, nonconfrontational, and requires the least trainer skill. We simply construct a narrow chute (with gates or with a sofa alongside a wall), toss a treat in, and wait for the dog to walk in and back out. **Molding** is the technique of using a prop to elicit the behavior.

Although not necessary from a conditioning perspective, the steps on this page utilize a touch pad at the end of the chute.

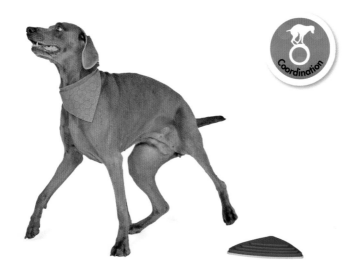

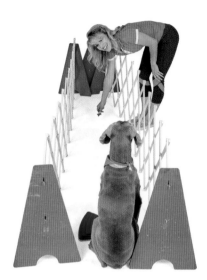

① Construct a chute that is narrow enough so that your dog cannot turn around in it. Show her as you drop a treat at the end.

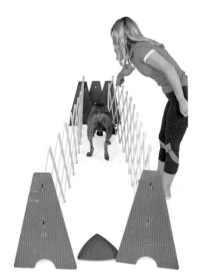

② Say "get it!" and let her go.

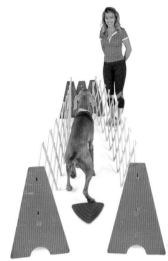

③ She will back out. She wants to see your face, so she will be more likely to back out and not turn around if you at the end of the chute.

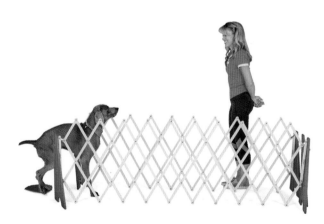

④ Put a touch pad (page 82) at the start of the chute. When your dog backs out, she will accidentally step on it. The moment she does, say "good!" and give her a treat. In this way, we are teaching her the useful targeting skill backing up to a touch pad.

Side-Step Drill

TECHNIQUE: LURING, BODY PRESSURE

BENEFITS: IMPROVES HIND END AWARENESS, STRENGTHENS INNER THIGH MUSCLES

In the **side-step drill** your dog keeps his front feet confined on something small and rotates his hind end around it. This exercise is sometimes called the elephant circle, as it mimics the routine of circus elephants on their pedestals.

There are two ways to get the dog to circle. One is with gentle body pressure, by using your leg to crowd in on his space, and the other is by using a treat to guide your dog to stay opposite of you. Often a combination of the two works best.

Do this exercise in both directions. Your dog will have a weaker side; work that side more.

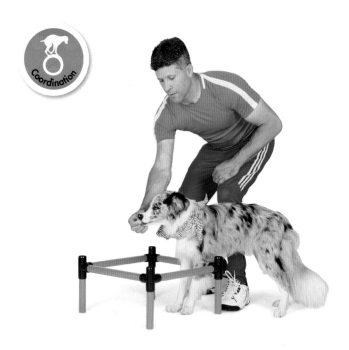

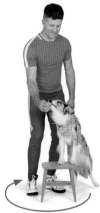 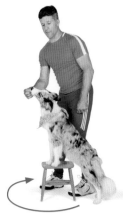 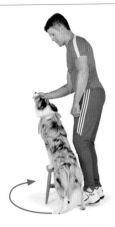

1. Lure your dog to put his front paws on a small, stable object (a taller object will be easier). Use a treat to keep your dog's head and front paws over the stool. Use your leg to crowd his space and cause him to shuffle over, circling his back feet around the stool.

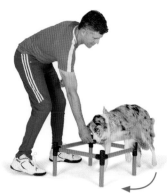 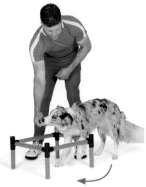 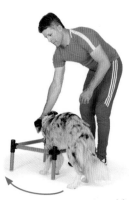

2. Try the side step drill with your dog's paws at ground level. Have him put his front paws in a Magic Square or in a bucket. Again, use a treat to hold his front end and your leg to bump his hind end.

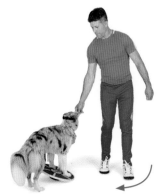 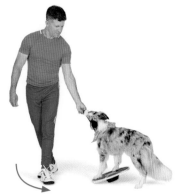

3. Combine the side step drill with a wobble board for added difficulty. Remember to work both directions.

Rainbow Ladder: Back Paws Only

TECHNIQUE:	LATERAL MOVEMENT
BENEFIT:	IMPROVE PROPRIOCEPTION/HIND-END AWARENESS

In level 2, your dog practiced **lateral movement** by sidestepping his front paws through the ladder rungs.

Even more challenging, your dog will now practice sidestepping his rear feet through the rungs.

REPEAT: 3–4 times on each side

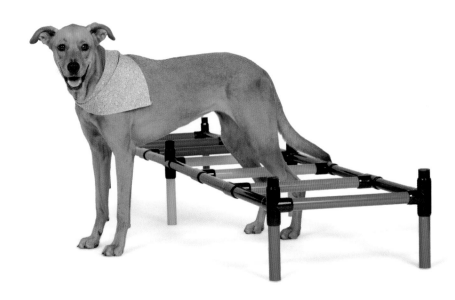

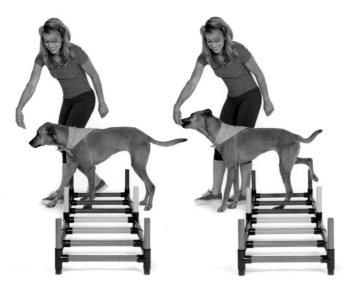

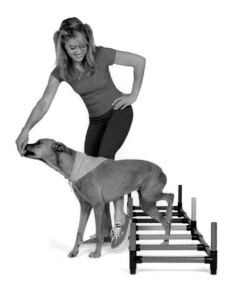

1. Set your ladder at a low height. The easiest way to get your dog's back feet in the ladder is to walk him all the way through, stopping when only his back feet remain.

2. Keep your dog's head engaged with a treat, and use your leg to body-pressure his hind end to sidestep.

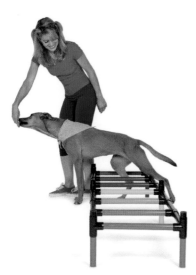

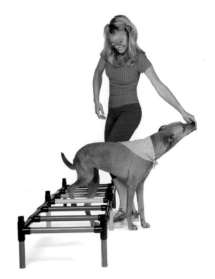

3. Raise the ladder height. This will be significantly more difficult for your dog, so move slowly. It may help to use your free hand to nudge his rear end.

4. Practice sidestepping both left and right. Your dog will be have a harder time in one direction; practice that side more.

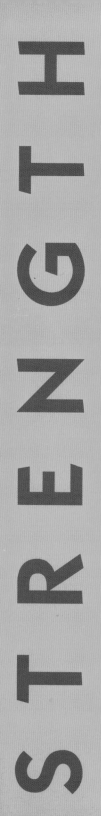

We all agree on the benefits of exercise, but how to we **motivate** our dog to actually do them?

With humans, we stay motivated to train with tricks like a favorite music playlist or a goal taped to our mirror. Most of our human motivational tricks won't translate into the dog world, but a few will.

- Motivate your dog with your "happy voice." Energy is contagious!

- Make a buddy system with your dog. Use the session to accomplish exercise goals for the both of you.

- Dogs are competitive. If your dog is slacking, set him aside and let him watch the fun you are having with another dog.

- Plan your workout schedule to coincide with times that your dog is naturally energetic; usually early mornings and early evenings.

- Dogs like routine. Work out at the same time of day, and structure your session consistently.

- This is your dog's one-on-one time with his favorite person—you! Be in the moment with him.

- Treats

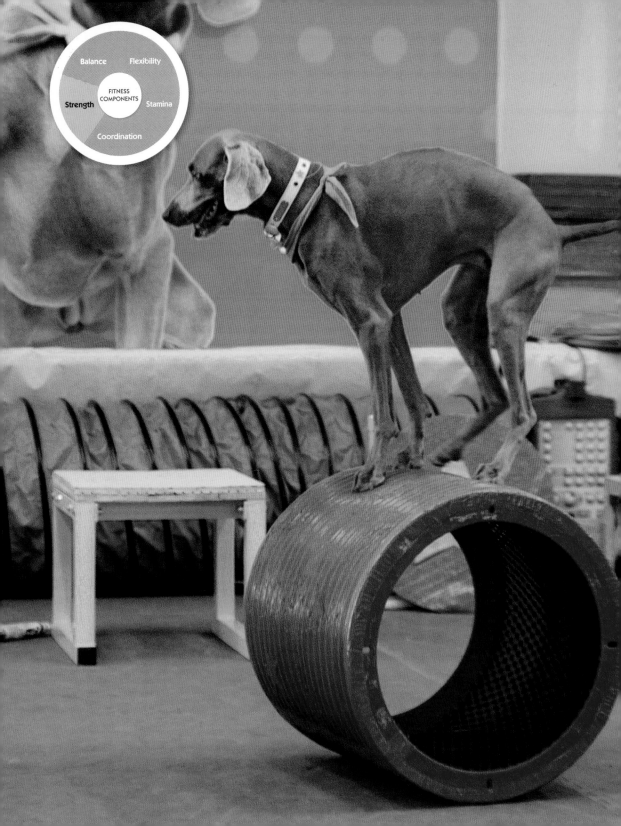

Balance   Flexibility

FITNESS
COMPONENTS

Strength   Stamina

Coordination

Neck: Push a Fit Ball

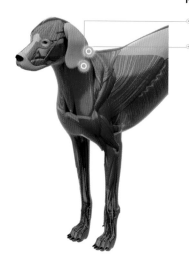

TECHNIQUE:	RESISTANCE TRAINING
BENEFIT:	STRENGTHENING OF NECK EXTENSION MUSCLES

In level 2 your dog exercised neck strength by pushing a **carpet roll** (page 92). This exercise is similar but with a greater **range of motion** and greater power.

This exercise specifically targets those muscles used in holding the dog's head up: his splenius muscle (at back of his neck) and his brachiocephalic muscle (at the sides of his neck).

NECK STRENGTHENING

⊙ Brachiocephalic muscle

⊙ Splenius muscle

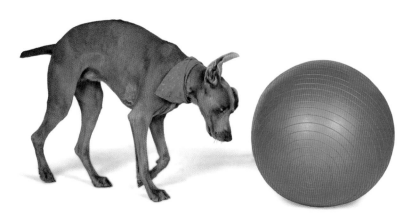

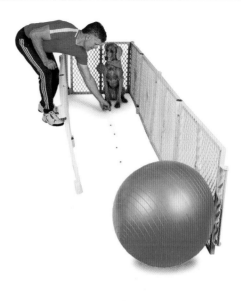

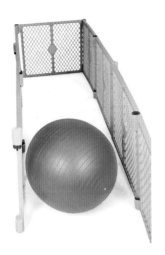

1 Construct a chute for your fit ball. A chute can be a sofa placed near the wall or a line of picnic benches near a wall.

2 Place a line of kibble or treats, and put the fit ball near your dog.

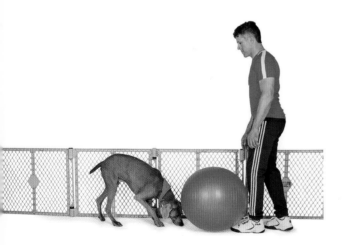

3 As your dog reaches for the first treat, she will push the ball forward and another treat will be revealed. If your dog is strong, fill the fit ball with a little water or sand to make it heavier.

Sit up High

STRENGTH

TECHNIQUE: MODELING

BENEFIT: STRENGTHENS ABDOMINAL AND EPAXIAL (BACK) MUSCLES

Active, athletic dogs benefit from core strengthening exercises to help prevent back injury. Older, arthritic dogs use core muscles to take stress off of their hind and front legs.

Strive for good posture, with the head forward and not pointed up, the back straight, and a square sit. Smaller dogs will have an easier time sitting up high, and not all dogs will be able to achieve this exercise. Improper posture can cause serious injuries, and any dog with neuro or spinal injuries should not do this exercise.

MODELING
When we use a treat to guide our dog into position, it is called **luring**. When we use our hands to guide or hold her in position, it is called **modeling**.

In this exercise, we use both techniques simultaneously.

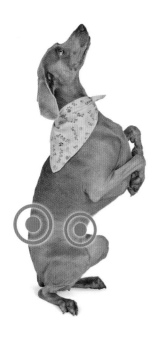

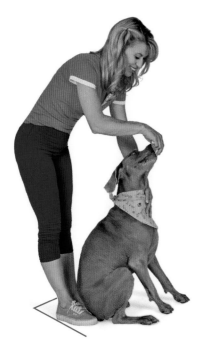
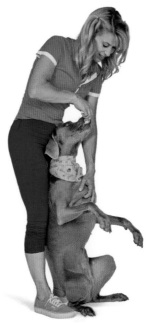
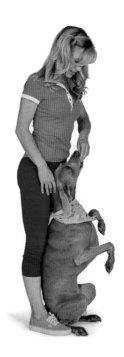

1 Have your dog sit squarely. Make a V with your feet, behind your dog. Lure her head up with one hand, and support her chest with the other.

2 Let her keep nibbling the treat while you support her. Many dogs (especially large breeds) will not have the core strength or balance to hold this position on their own.

3 After many short training sessions, your dog will have the core strength to support herself, but will still rely on your legs for balance.

Roll Over

TECHNIQUE: GYMNASTIC

BENEFIT: STRENGTHENS CORE MUSCLES

Gymnastic is a physical exercise designed to develop strength and coordination. A roll over requires explosive strength, utilizing the dog's core. This exercise will be harder for some body types than others.

It can be helpful to first train a roll over on a slight incline, such as a slightly sloped backyard. With your dog parallel to the slope, he need only roll onto his back and gravity will take him the rest of the way over.

In level 2, your dog learned a **lying neck stretch** (page 62). Roll over begins with that same neck stretch and continues it farther.

SIGNS OF A WEAK CORE

• Poor posture such as a swayback topline

• Poor balance, such as standing on three legs when you support the fourth

• Excessive sway in back-end movement

• Difficulty transitioning from positions such as sitting to standing

• Inability to hold a sit or stand for long

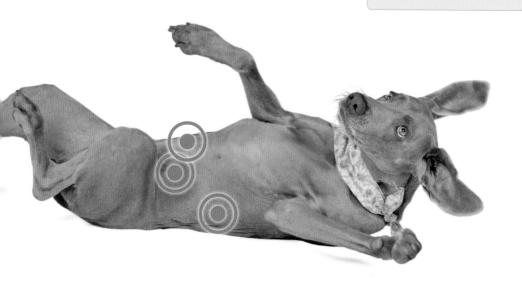

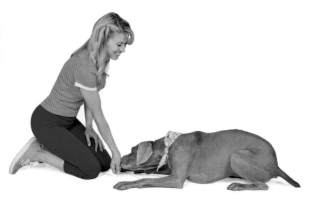

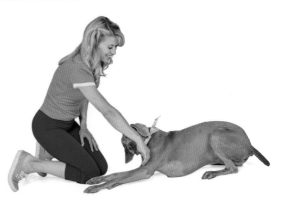

1. Hold several small treats in your hand. Hold your hand to your dog's nose to get her interest.

2. Notice if your dog is already laying on one haunch or the other and plan your roll in that direction. Move the treat to your dog's shoulder.

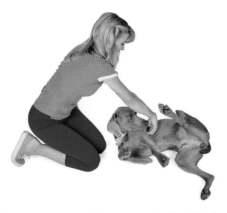

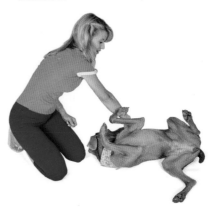

3. From her shoulder, move the treat to her backbone. You can give her small treats along the way.

4. Continue moving the treat to the floor. If she stalls out, you can gently guide her front legs over (although some dogs balk at this).

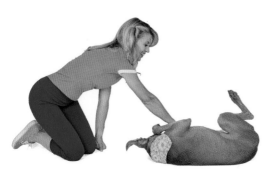

5. Give her another treat at the end. Dogs will have a weaker side. Work that direction more.

Assisted Upright Walking

TECHNIQUE: BODY WEIGHT

BENEFIT: STRENGTHENS CORE, FRONT AND HIND END/IMPROVES FLEXIBILITY IN HIP FLEXORS (ILIOPSOAS)

In level 2, your dog learned to put his **paws on your arm** (page 94). We will now build on that skill by having your dog use your arm for support while he walks forward, upright.

This exercise takes considerable strength in your dog's core, as well as both his hind limbs and his forelimbs. It's a full body workout. This exercise will take strength on your part, as well.

BENEFITS OF A STRONG CORE

- Improves posture

- Maintains balance

- Supports the back muscles, which in turn supports the entire body

- Decreases incidence of injuries associated with osteoarthritis and other soft tissue issues

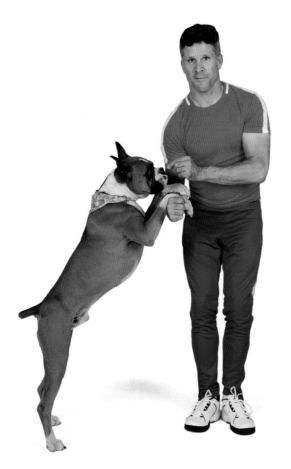

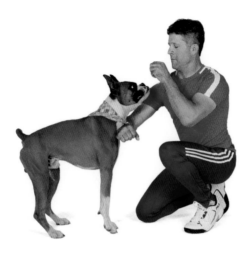

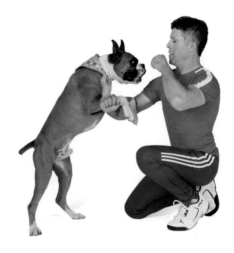

1. Start kneeling down. Make sure your arm is steady, to give your dog the confidence to lean on it.

2. Use a treat to lure his paws on your arm. Alternately, you can scoop up his paws with your arm.

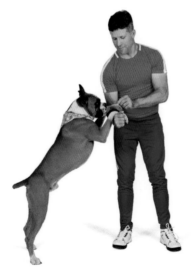

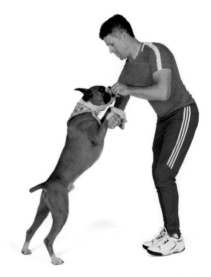

3. Stand up, keeping your dog's interest with a few treats.

4. Walk backwards, causing your dog to walk forward. Give him a treat every few seconds to keep him motivated.

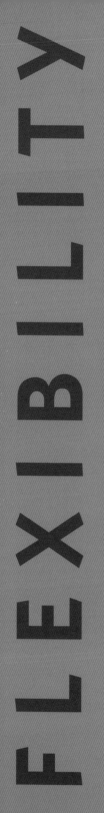

FLEXIBILITY

In previous levels we trained with **static stretching** and **dynamic stretching**. Recently, coaches of human athletes have started leaning toward functional stretching as a primary technique for improving the flexibility of their athletes.

Functional flexibility should be based on the specific task of the canine athlete's sport, and it should provide stability and strength that matches the full range of motion of that task.

To use a human example, if an athlete is looking to improve functional flexibility for golf, his functional flexibility exercise would resemble a golf swing. The exercise should create a similar reaction in his foot, knee, hip, and shoulder to what would occur in golf. The exercise takes the athlete through the entire range of motion, at a controlled speed.

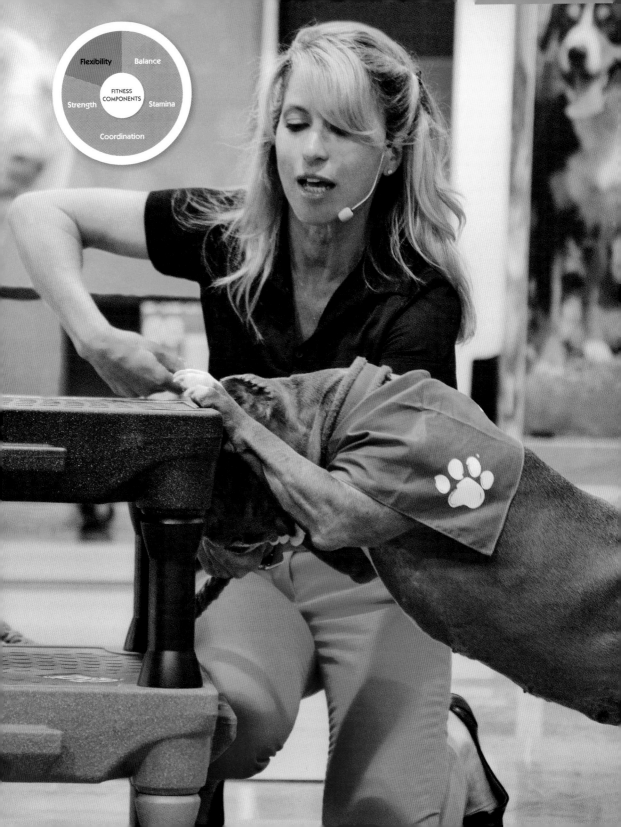

FITNESS COMPONENTS

Flexibility

Balance

Strength

Stamina

Coordination

2-on/2-off Extreme Bow

TECHNIQUE:	DYNAMIC STRETCHING
BENEFIT:	IMPROVES FLEXIBILITY IN SHOULDERS, HIP FLEXORS (ILIOPSOAS), AND EXPAXIAL MUSCLES

Dynamic stretching warm-ups are standard routine in the sports world as an effective method for athletes to prep before an event.

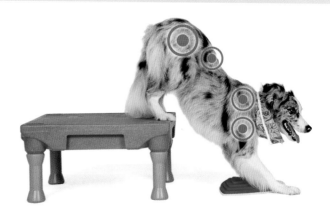

Dynamic stretching is a walking or movement stretch, where the dog is moving as he stretches (like walking lunges in human stretching). By performing slow, controlled movements through full range of motion, the risk of injury is reduced.

Dynamic stretching improves range of motion and body awareness. It challenges the dog's balance and coordination; skills that could help his performance.

Have your dog warm up before this exercise as it works multiple muscles.

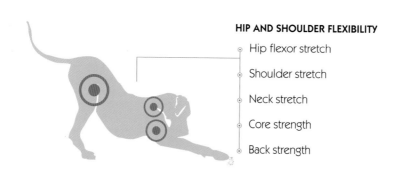

HIP AND SHOULDER FLEXIBILITY

- Hip flexor stretch
- Shoulder stretch
- Neck stretch
- Core strength
- Back strength

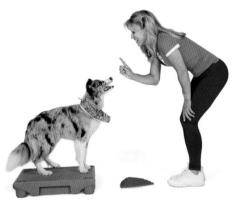

① Start with your dog on a low platform in front of a touch target.

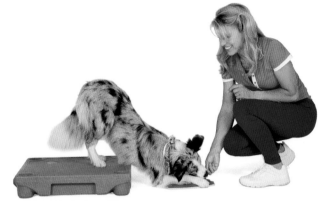

② Lure your dog to touch the target. Keep the treat low, near the target. He should go into a bow. If he lies down, put your hand under his belly.

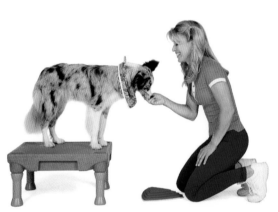

③ Now use a higher platform. Start with the lure at your dog's nose.

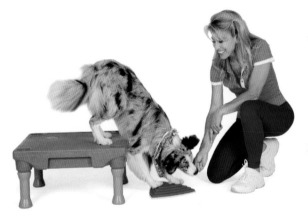

④ The placement of the target will affect the stretch angle of his shoulders and hips.

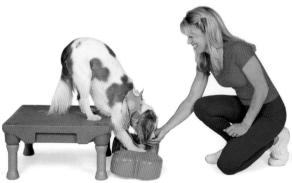

⑤ As a variation, use an unstable object such as a fit bone for the target.

Slant Board Swimmer's Turn

TECHNIQUE: FUNCTIONAL FLEXIBILITY

BENEFIT: IMPROVES AGILITY/STRENGTHENS HIND AND FORE LIMBS

In the sport of **flyball**, a dog runs to a slanted board, grabs a ball, and switches direction to run back. It's not good to have a dog jam into the boar, hard, with his forelimbs so, instead, we teach dogs to do a swimmer's turn. In a swimmer's turn, the dog does a fluid circle on the slant board, with a low-impact change of direction.

In this **functional flexibility** exercise, we take the dog through the entire range of motion at a slower, more controlled speed.

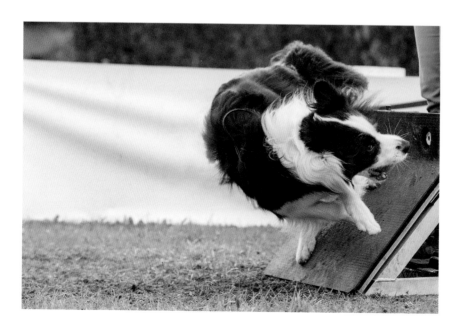

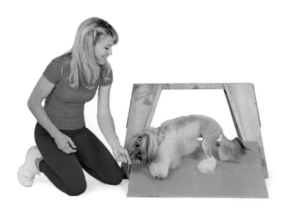

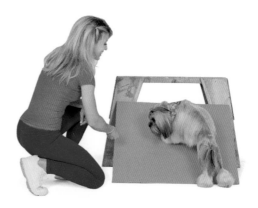

1. Start with a very low incline on your board. Have your dog follow a treat in a circle. Traction surface will help. Try adding a rubber mat, carpet, or traction spray.

2. Set the board at a steeper incline. Your dog will need a running start to bank the turn; use your voice to motivate him.

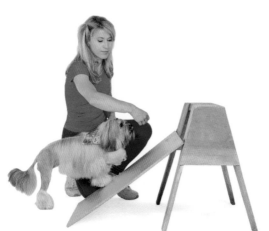

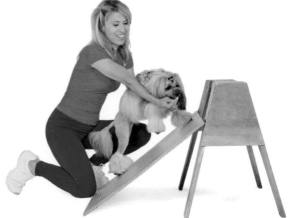

3. Keep your lure at the dog's nose height and take him in a wide circle.

4. Try to take your dog in a fluid circle, where all four paws are on the slant board at once.

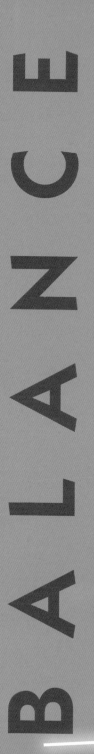

BALANCE

Balancing has been proven to have cognitive benefits, including memory, in humans, especially for seniors.

Balance training will boost the power of your dog's brain by engaging the nervous system to take on new challenges. Each balance exercise is a riddle for your dog's brain and body to figure out. Your dog must learn which muscles to activate, with how much force, and at what time.

At first, your dog will struggle to maintain balance on a teeter-totter. After doing it often, however, it will eventually become easy; your dog will have sprouted new neural connections and muscle memory to be able to maneuver this prop with ease. Your dog's brain is involved just as much as his limbs.

Giving your dog a variety of new balance challenges will maximize the cognitive benefits.

While some dogs are naturally gifted at balance, others are not. The good news is that balance can be significantly improved with practice!

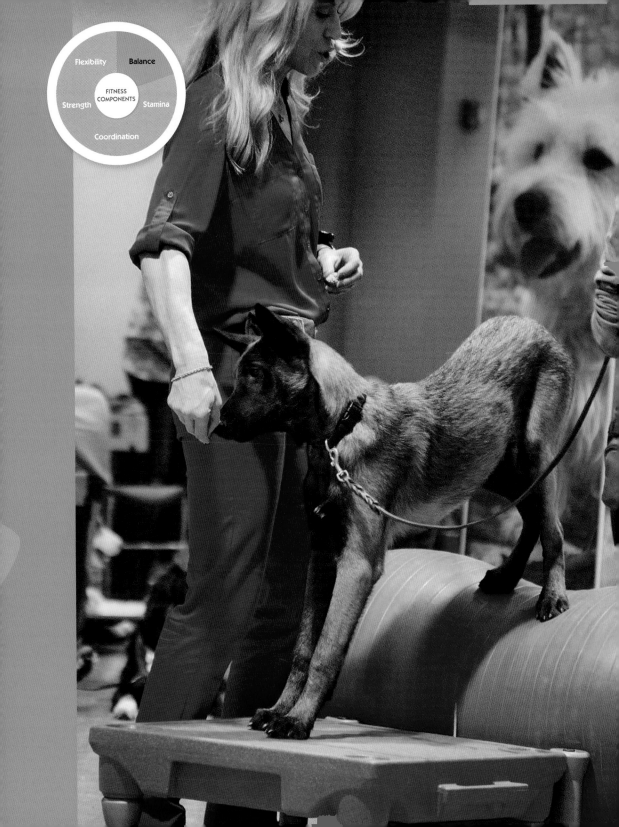

Flexibility Balance

FITNESS
COMPONENTS

Strength Stamina

Coordination

Moon Bounce Peanuts

TECHNIQUE:	INSTABILITY TRAINING
BENEFIT:	IMPROVES BALANCE, OVERALL BODY STRENGTHENING

Balance work enables you to target postural muscles and reflexes. These are muscles that help hold your dog up against gravity. Balance exercises work the whole body with the contraction of many muscle groups from the shoulders and forelimbs, all the way down the spine and core, to the hips and hind legs.

Instead of repetitions, in balance exercises we gauge in duration, or how long can the dog can sustain the exercise. Start with a few minutes at a time and observe your dog's tolerance.

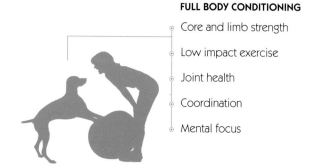

FULL BODY CONDITIONING

- Core and limb strength
- Low impact exercise
- Joint health
- Coordination
- Mental focus

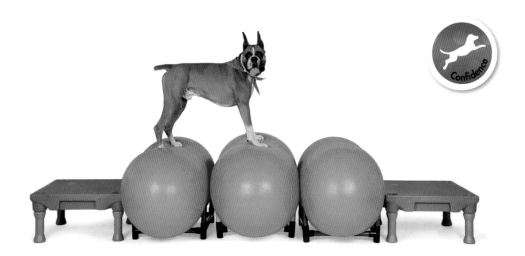

Confidence

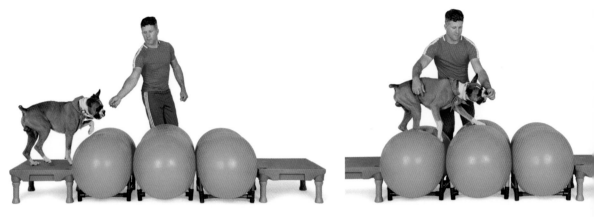

1. Place a step at the entrance and exit of the moon bounce, to keep movements slow and controlled.

2. Allow your dog to control the action, but keep your hand on his body for safety.

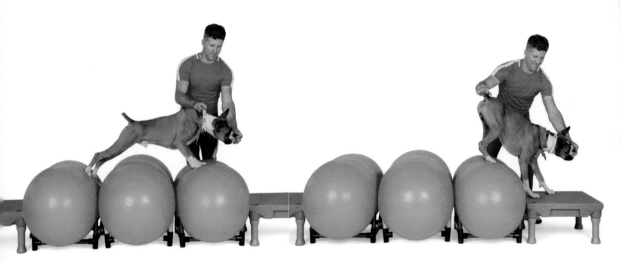

3. It is not important how your dog chooses to maneuver the peanuts. So long as he is struggling to balance, he is being strengthened.

4. Carefully control the exit, as this is the part most at risk for sporadic movement and injury.

Teeter-Totter

TECHNIQUE:	DYNAMIC BALANCE
BENEFIT:	IMPROVES DYNAMIC BALANCE, STRENGTHENS FORE LIMBS

The teeter-totter is an extension of the **balance beam** exercise (page 74) that your dog learned in level 2. This exercise is different from all of the other exercises, in that it has a tipping point, which can be startling at first for a dog.

It is not uncommon for novice dogs have a startling experience with a teeter-totter and immediately develop a fear of it. The fear can be overcome, but it could take months. Instead, introduce this piece of exercise equipment to your dog slowly and control its movement at all times to keep it steady.

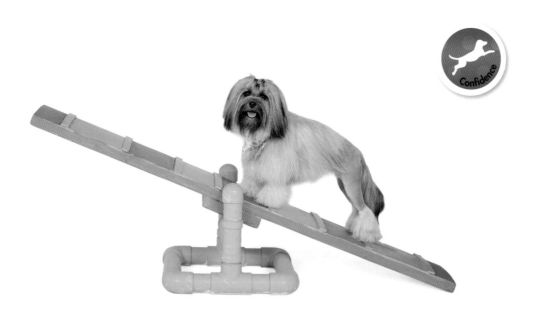

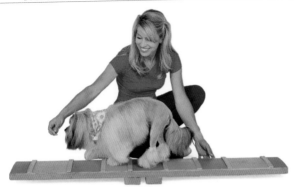

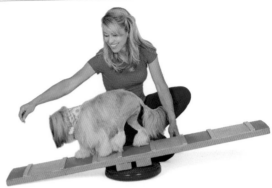

1. Set the board on the ground and lure your dog to step on it. Set it on a pencil or small beam to give it a tiny bit of rock.

2. Set the board on a balance disc.

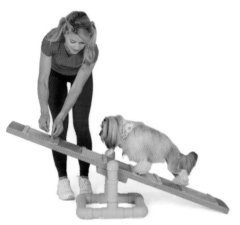

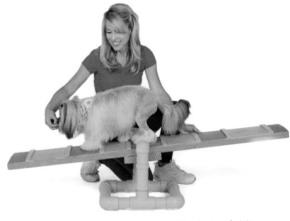

3. Ready to go higher? Lay a line of treats along the board for your dog to follow.

4. Control the board at the tipping point to prevent it from slamming down.

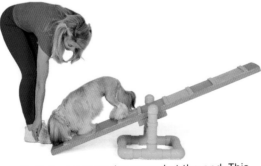

5. Set a treat on the ground at the end. This habituates your dog to slowing down at the end instead of leaping off.

Balance on a Block

TECHNIQUE: SMALL-STANCE BALANCE

BENEFIT: IMPROVES BALANCE/STRENGTHENS STABILIZER MUSCLES/IMPROVES PROPRIOCEPTION

This advanced skill requires intense mental focus and strong toes, wrists, and ankles.

Balance is easier in a wide stance, with all four feet spread apart. By confining the feet into a small box, the dog must be very precise in positioning his body weight at the center.

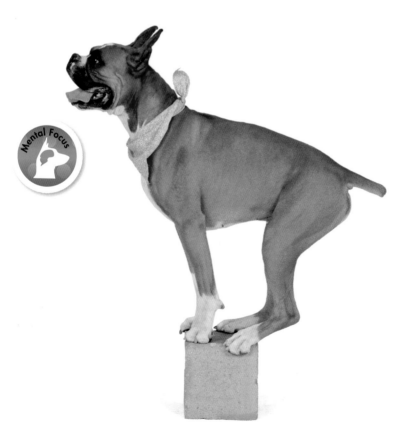

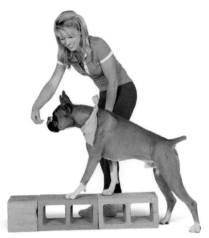

1 Set a row of cement blocks, and lure your dog to walk the beam.

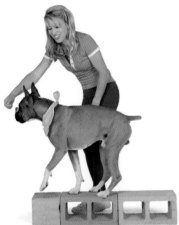

2 Use your knee to body block him from one side, and maybe a wall to block the other side.

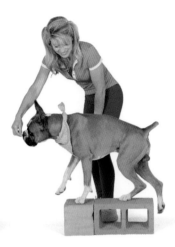

3 Remove one block.

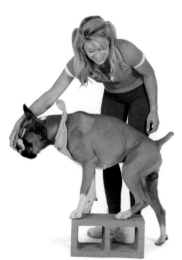

4 Remove another block. Tap his back leg to prompt in onto the block.

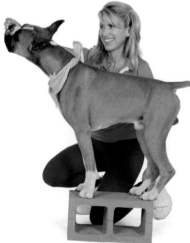

5 Let him nibble a treat when he is in the correct position.

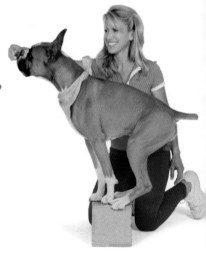

6 You may have to help him get all four paws on the small block. Tap or left each paw that comes off.

STAMINA

In humans, endurance energy is mostly generated from glucose (sugar) from glycogen stores. This is why marathon runners carbo-load and ingest gel packs (sugar) during the race. Dogs, by contrast, use **fat** as energy for endurance exercise. High-carbohydrate diets are not ideal for performance dogs, as they reduce stamina.

For more optimized performance, a working dog's diet should contain a highly digestible source of fat and protein to prepare his muscles and metabolism for exercise, as well as provide energy that is readily available for exercise.

Canine athletes should be fed a high-fat, high-protein diet to help maximize training and conditioning. A diet high in fat and protein can help boost a dog's metabolism and endurance.

It is not recommended to feed canine athletes before strenuous, intensive exercise. In most cases, a dog should be fed at least 60 minutes after exercise or 10 to 12 hours before exercise. Ideally, a dog should be fed the night before exercise the next morning, as complete digestion takes 20 to 24 hours.

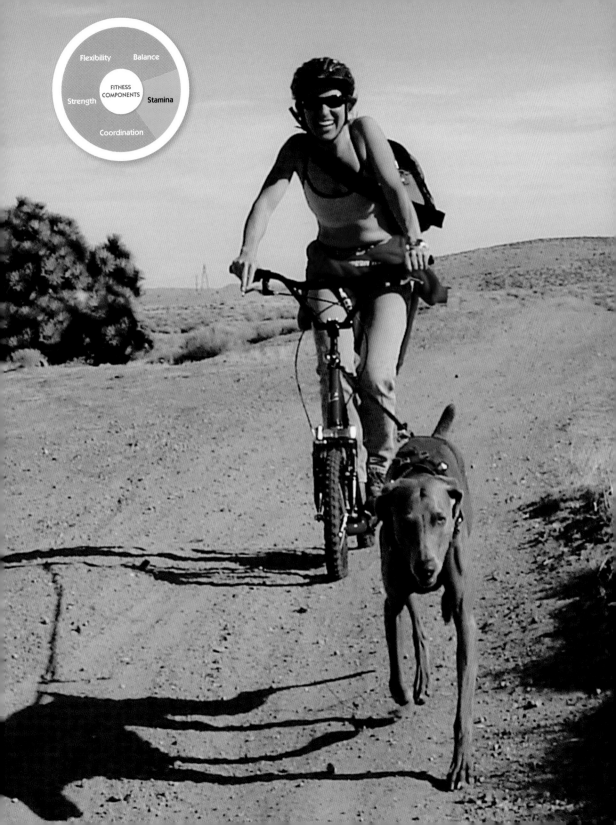

FITNESS
COMPONENTS

Flexibility   Balance

Strength   Stamina

Coordination

Scootering

STAMINA

TECHNIQUE:	CARDIO
BENEFIT:	IMPROVES ENDURANCE AND MUSCLE STAMINA

This sport is similar to the **weight pull** exercise in level 2.

Dog mushing can be done in a variety of ways; on snow with a sled or on skis, or on a wheeled land cart or scooter. It can be done with one or multiple dogs. Dogs may need to start with a weight less than the weight of a person, and some dogs may never be able to easily pull that weight.

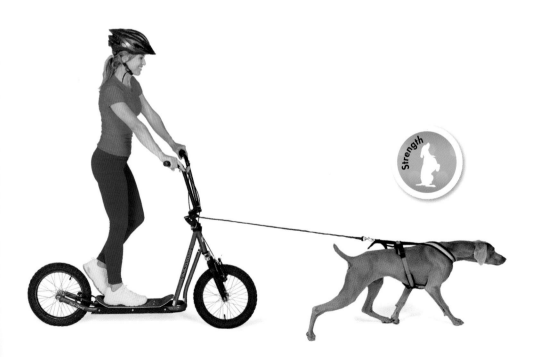

Strength

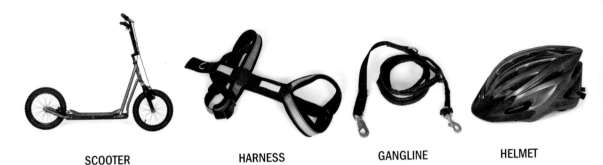

SCOOTER   HARNESS   GANGLINE   HELMET

1 A dog scooter is heavy duty with wider dirt tires. A mushing harness is long, with the O-ring attachment near the dog's tail. The gangline has a bungee portion to absorb shock. Falls are part of the sport, so wear your helmet.

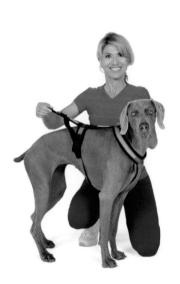

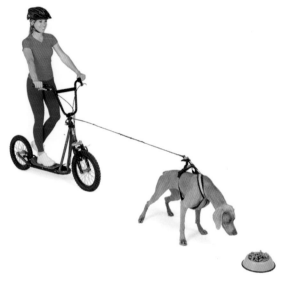

2 Use a specially designed dog-mushing harness with padding and an attachment point near the base of the tail.

3 There are several tactics to entice a dog to pull. You can start by having her pull toward a food bowl. Dogs are competitive in mushing, and having another person or dog act as a "rabbit" for them to chase is very effective.

COORDINATION

In previous levels, the coordination exercises were relatively straightforward; walking through cavalettis, jumping, circling, and targeting. In level 4, we are going to challenge our dog to not just go in instinct but to work thoughtfully, thinking through each foot placement.

These skills are not ones that we can merely lure or guide a dog through. These skill require trainer skill to communicate the task to the dog, and they require a dog versed in training who is an active participant in the learning process.

Coordination task are usually fun for a dog (they are for humans, as well!) Unsteady and clumsy at first, with practice, the dog learns to isolate each foot and easily and quickly place it where it belongs. The **double-rail balance beam** is one that you may find your dog hopping on all by himself, just for fun.

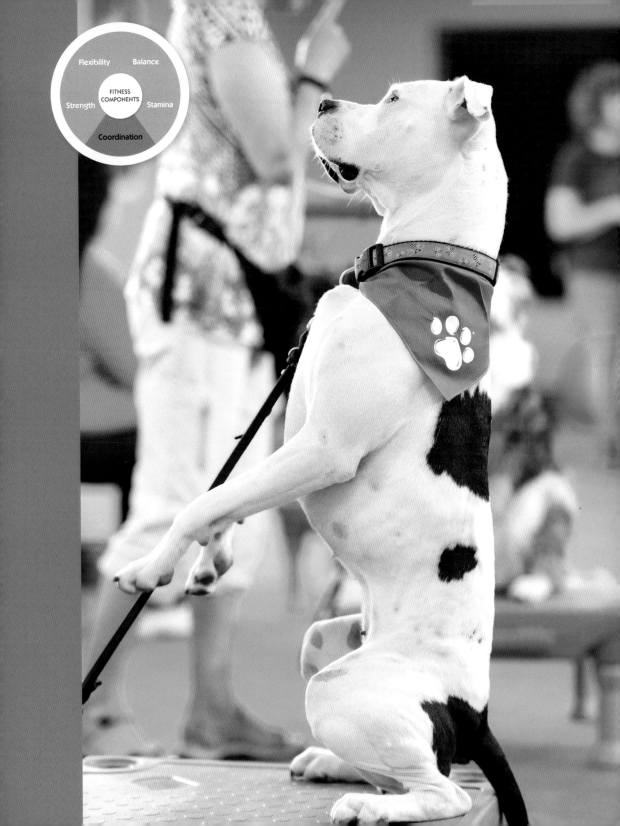

FITNESS COMPONENTS

Flexibility   Balance

Strength   Stamina

Coordination

Rear Leg Hike

TECHNIQUE:	COORDINATION ISOLATION
BENEFIT:	STRENGTHENS HIP FLEXORS (ILIOPSOAS)

Dogs' limbs generally move on a parallel plane, and not to the side. In the **leg hike** exercise, we challenge our dog to **isolate** one rear limb and to lift it to the side.

It is harder for a dog to think in the abstract about lifting a rear leg than it is for her to think about placing her rear leg on an object. We teach leg hike by rewarding our dog for rear-foot touching an increasing stack of touch pads.

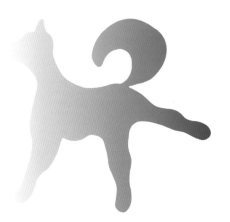

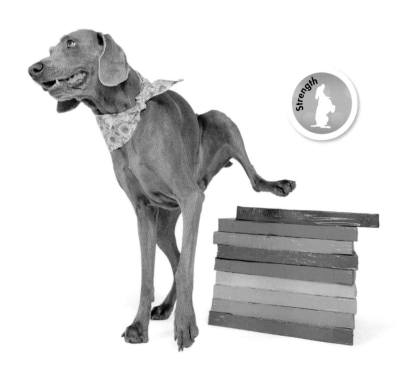

Strength

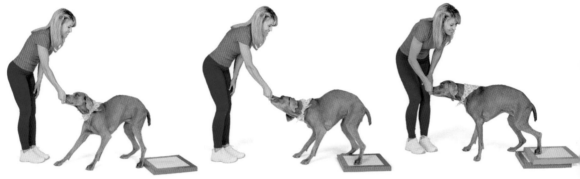

1. Start with your dog a few inches (5 cm) in front of a touch pad. At nose height, push a treat towards her, causing her to back up.

2. The instant one foot touches the touch pad, say "good!" and release the treat. Timing is crucial.

3. After about 10 successes, add a second touch pad.

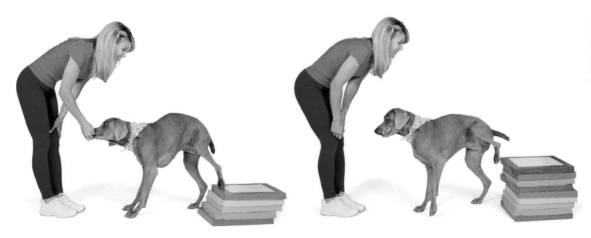

4. Continue to add touch pads. Keep the treat at nose height as a high neck would make balance and flexibility more difficult.

5. Eventually, by continually marking the moment with "good!" and giving a treat, your dog will understand the concept and be able to do the behavior without the treat at her nose.

Barrel Roll: 4 Feet

COORDINATION

TECHNIQUE:	DYNAMIC SMALL STANCE BALANCE
BENEFIT:	STRENGTHENS CORE AND LEG MUSCLES/IMPROVES MENTAL FOCUS

This advanced skill combines the previously learned skills of **rolling a barrel with two feet** (page 120) and **balancing on a small block** (page 150).

The dog will walk forward on top of the barrel, moving each foot one at a time. All four feet are constricted into a small space, making balance hard. By adding a rolling barrel, this small stance balance becomes dynamic and even harder.

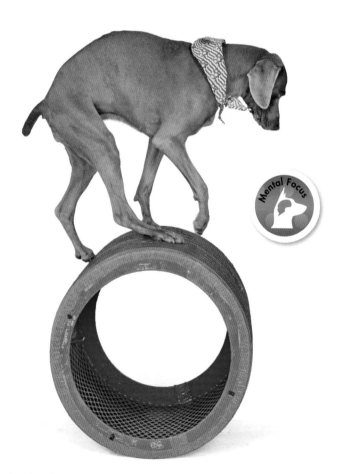

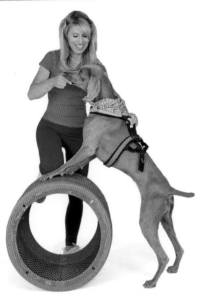 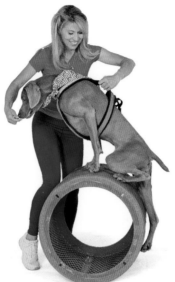 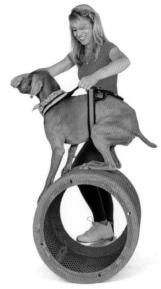

① A harness will be helpful. Always keep a knee or foot on the barrel to steady it.

② Use a treat to lure your dog onto the barrel. Keep her steady by holding her harness with your other hand.

③ Once up, help her find her balance point. When she is ready to dismount, have her walk forward and off.

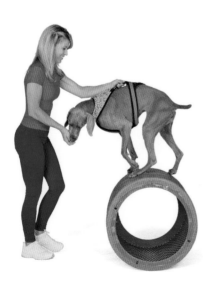 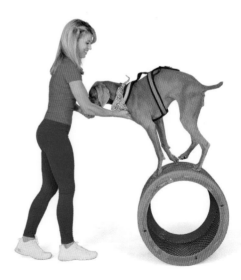

④ Stand in front of your dog. Keep control of her while you walk forward. This will cause her feet to walk forward.

⑤ As she improves, let go of her harness and instead use a treat to hold her on the barrel, and use your other hand to push into her chest.

Side-Step Drill: Ball/Disc

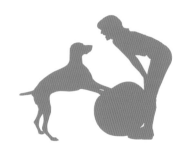

TECHNIQUE: BODY PRESSURE

BENEFITS: IMPROVES HIND END AWARENESS/STRENGTHENS FORELIMB MUSCLES THAT STABILIZE WRISTS

In level 3, your dog learned the **side-step drill** (page 124) by circling with his front feet on a stool or confined inside a Magic Square.

In this exercise, we will increase the difficulty by having your dog circle with his front feet on a ball or confined inside a flying disc.

As before, we can get the dog to circle by using a treat to keep his head in place and using gentle body pressure to crowd his space and get him to side step.

Do this exercise in both directions. Your dog will have a weaker side; work that side more.

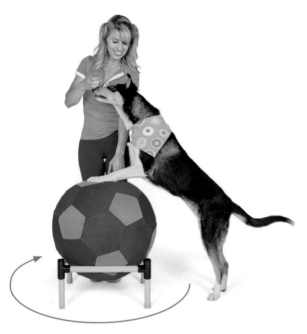

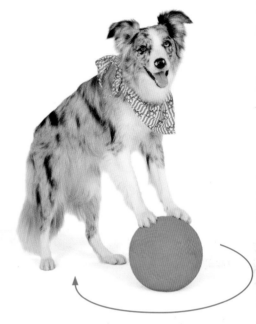

1 Stabilize a fit ball inside a Magic Square. Center your dog's head by holding a treat above the ball. Side step into your dog to get him to shuffle his back feet around the ball.

2 For smaller dogs, use a playground ball stabilized in a dog food bowl. With very good balance, your dog can learn to side step on an unstabilized ball.

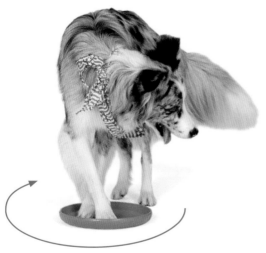

3 Some dogs can side step with a flying disc. Place it upside down on the carpet. Your dog's front paws remain stationary, and the disc rotates on top of the carpet as your dog side steps.

Balance Beam: Double Rail

TECHNIQUE: PRECISION FOOT PLACEMENT

BENEFIT: IMPROVES PROPRIOCEPTION AND COORDINATION ISOLATION

The **double-rail balance beam** is one that dogs really enjoy! The dog walks with her right feet on one beam and left feet on the other.

Make a double rail beam with 2" x 4" (2 cm x 4 cm) wood beams. If you find your dog is continually jumping off the beams, you may need to raise them higher.

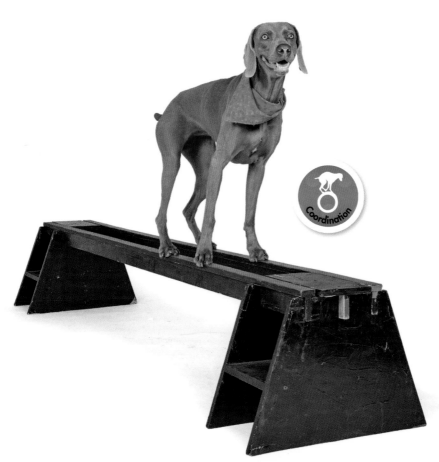

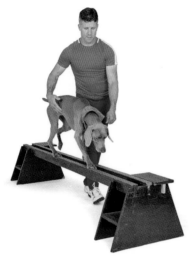

1 Start with the two beams touching or close together so that they resemble a solid plank.

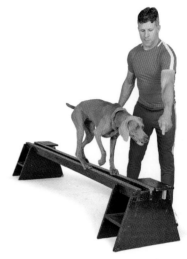

2 Control your dog all the way to the end, as dogs often leap off prematurely.

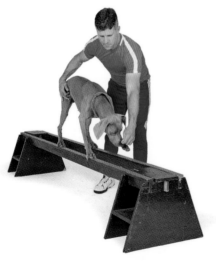

3 Spread the beams apart. Hold a treat in your front hand, low to the beams. Use your back hand to guard your dog's body, in case she starts to lose balance.

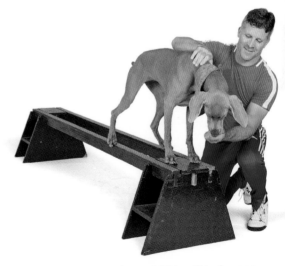

4 Give a treat at the end. This will train your dog to stop at that point.

Rainbow Ladder: Step Backward

TECHNIQUE: LATERAL MOVEMENT

BENEFIT: IMPROVE PROPRIOCEPTION/HIND-END AWARENESS

In level 2, your dog practiced **lateral movement** by sidestepping his front paws through the ladder rungs.

Even more challenging, your dog will now practice sidestepping his rear feet through the rungs.

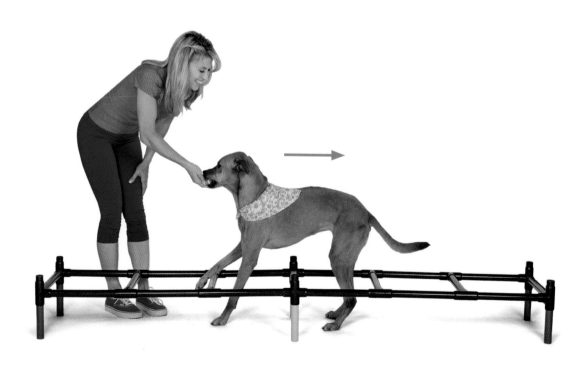

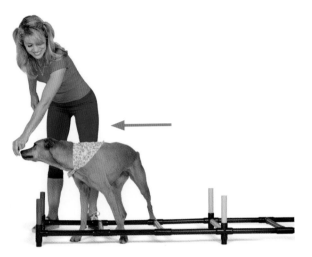

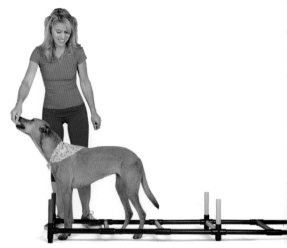

1 The easiest way to get all four of your dog's feet in the ladder is to walk him through forward.

2 Once all four feet are in, keep your dog's head engaged with a treat.

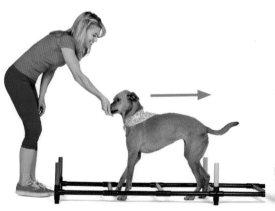

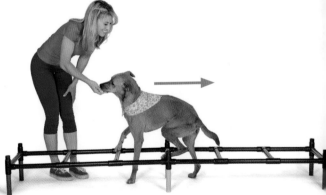

3 Holding the treat at your dog's nose height, slowly push it toward him, causing him to recoil his head and step backward.

4 A higher ladder will challenge your dog to high step as he walks backward.

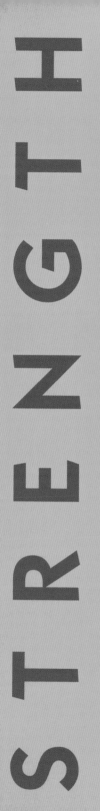
STRENGTH

Our dogs run, play, and chase on a regular basis—some more than others. This daily movement is good conditioning for their muscles and cardiovascular system, however, the biggest improvements are seen from exercises that "confuse" the muscles.

Muscle confusion is the idea that constantly varying workouts results in a more comprehensive workout where muscles are hit in many ways and get more positive benefits. By constantly switching up your dog's workout, he'll be training more of his muscles. A body is an adaptive machine; it's going to get better at handling whatever stress is put on it the more it does. So by stressing it in different ways, it has more chances to positively adapt.

In level 4, our dog will be trying some new and interesting challenges, including some **inverted exercises** where the dog is in a modified handstand.

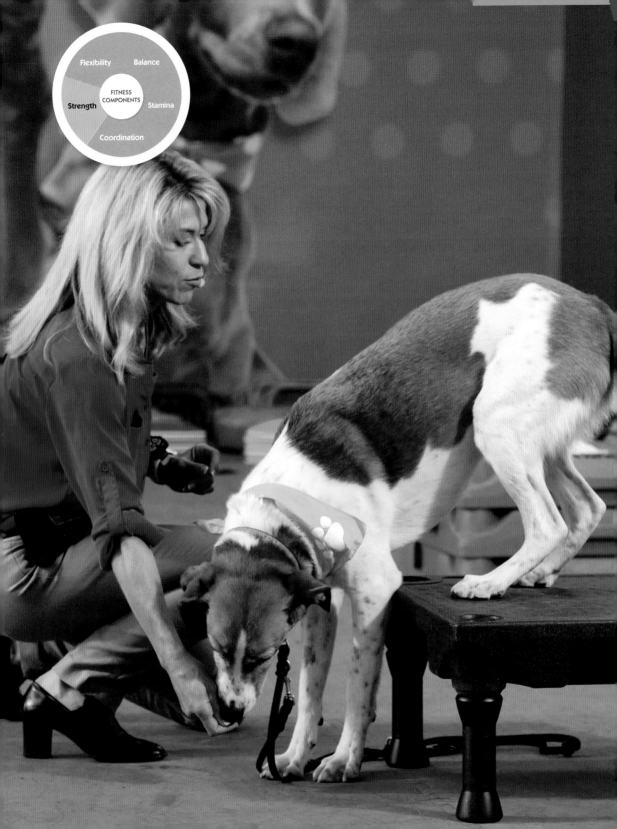

FITNESS COMPONENTS

Flexibility   Balance

Strength   Stamina

Coordination

2-on/2-off Pull Back on

TECHNIQUE: INVERTED EXERCISE

BENEFIT: STRENGTHENS CORE MUSCLES AND HIP FLEXORS (ILIOPSOAS)

In this exercise, we start with the previous skill of the **extreme bow** (page 140) and add on to it. Once our dog is in the bow position, we get him to use great strength in his core to pull his front feet back onto the platform.

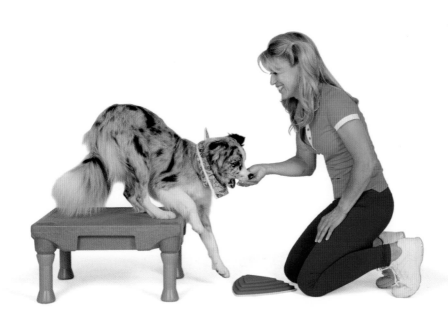

STEPS:

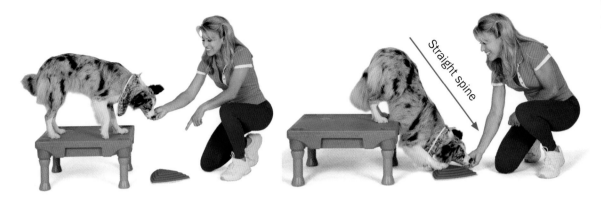

1. As in the extreme bow exercise, we start with the dog on a platform and a touch pad in front of him.

2. Slowly lure him down by putting a treat near the touch pad. Use your hand under his belly if he tries to lie down.

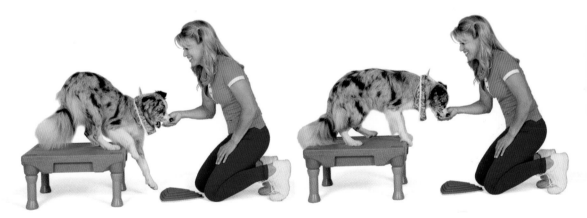

3. Lift the treat up and toward the platform. This should cause your dog to arch his neck and pull back onto the platform. Dogs sometimes lie down. This is not ideal, but it is still accomplishing some strength training.

4. Release the treat when your dog is in the correct position—on the platform.

Handstand

TECHNIQUE: INVERTED EXERCISE

BENEFIT: STRENGTHENS CORE, FRONT AND HIND LIMBS, HIP FLEXORS (ILIOPSOAS)

This technical exercise stresses your dog's flexibility as well as his core and limb strength.

In order to teach this exercise, we will use the same technique used for **rear leg hike** (page 158). We will push a treat in toward the dog, causing him to back up. The slant of the handstand board will increase.

The slant board should have traction; either a textured surface or wooden slats.

Depending on the dog's breed and physiology, he will be able to achieve only a certain height and angle of the board, with correct posture. Observe where your dog maxes out, and let that be your final objective.

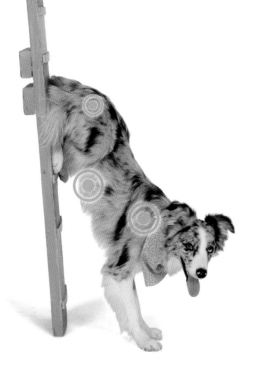

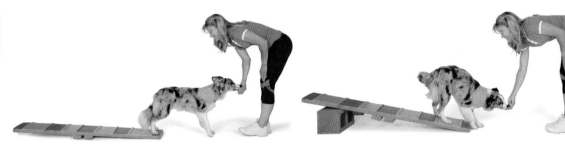

1. Start with your dog a few inches (5 cm) in front of the board. Hold a treat at his nose height, and push it toward him to cause him to back onto the board.

2. Incline the board by putting one end on a cement block.

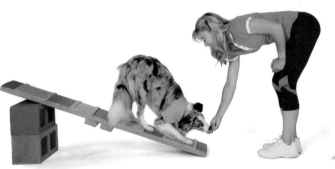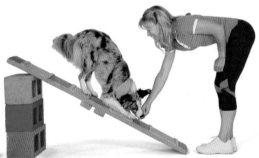

3. Increase the angle with another cement block. Always hold the treat low to the ground.

4. Add a third block. Have your dog back up a few feet (0.5 m). Keep the treat low, so he is not forced to arch his neck.

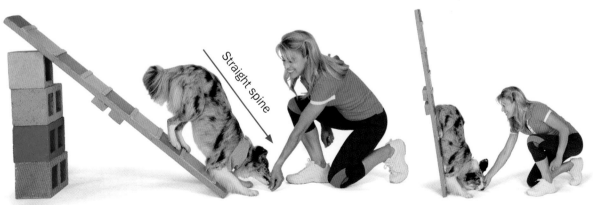

Straight spine

5. With a fourth block, your dog may no longer be able to get his front paws on the board. Keep your treat low to keep a straight spine.

6. Some dog body types can achieve a higher angle than others. Hold your treat in a spot that benefits your dog's balance.

Paw Swipe at Muzzle

TECHNIQUE: MOLDING

BENEFIT: STRENGTHENS CORE AND SHOULDER MUSCLES/IMPROVES BALANCE

We've previously taught our dog to **leg hike** (page 158) where we challenged him to isolate one rear limb and lift it to the side. In this exercise, our dog will train our dog to lift one front limb high to his muzzle. Not only does this work the dog's shoulder, but it works his core muscles, as well.

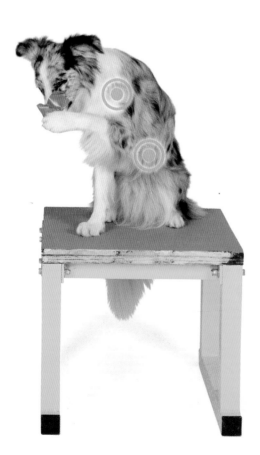

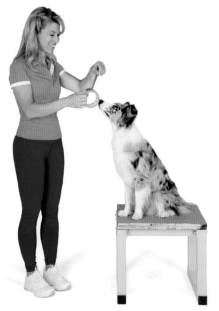

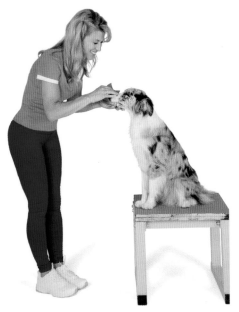

1. Use a piece of tape. Press it on your jeans a few times to make it less sticky.

2. Stick it on your dog's muzzle, preferably on the side that you wish him to lift his paw.

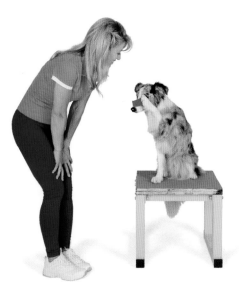

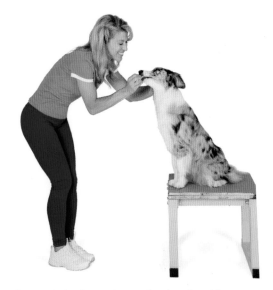

3. Your dog will lift his paw to swipe away the tape. Occasionally, dogs will lie down. Putting them on a platform will make this less likely.

4. Mark the instant your dog touches his muzzle by saying "good!" and immediately give him a treat.

PROFESSIONAL EXPERT REVIEWERS

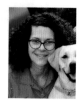

CINDY OTTO, DVM, PhD, DACVECC, DACVSMR
Director, Penn Vet Working Dog Center
As director of the Penn Vet Working Dog Center, one of Dr. Otto's major areas of research and practice is fitness, conditioning, and physical rehabilitation of working and sporting dogs. The PVWDC is a pioneer in the working dog field whose goal it is to increase collaborative research and the application of the newest scientific findings and veterinary expertise to optimize the performance of lifesaving detection dogs.

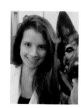

MEGHAN RAMOS, VMD
Dr. Ramos is a veterinarian and research fellow at the Penn Vet Working Dog Center for performance and working dogs. She began her master's degree in translational medicine through the University of Pennsylvania and will pursue a residency in Canine Sports Medicine and Rehabilitation.

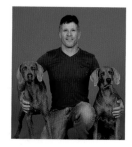

ROB CLARK
Rob and Kyra, together, have produced over 60 canine conditioning workshops and certified over a thousand Canine Conditioning Coaches. With a fitness and wellness background, and as an accomplished wrestler and football player, Rob is an advocate of physical activity for both humans and dogs. Rob enjoys being in nature and outdoor activities with his active dogs.

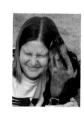

REGINA R. ALLEN, DVM
With a background as a veterinarian in small animal practice, Dr. Allen works as an adjunct professor at Laurel Highlands Community College and instructs on competition dog sports.